D1365807

Choice, Control and Contemporary Childbirth

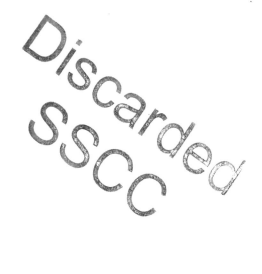

Choice, Control and Contemporary Childbirth

UNDERSTANDING THROUGH WOMEN'S STORIES

JULIE JOMEEN

PhD, MSc, RM, RGN
Senior Lecturer in Midwifery
University of Hull

Foreword by

TINA LAVENDER

Professor of Midwifery
University of Manchester

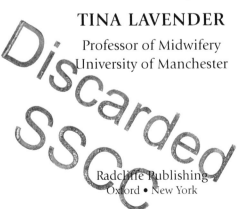

Radcliffe Publishing
Oxford • New York

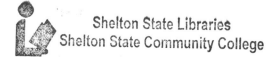

Radcliffe Publishing Ltd
18 Marcham Road
Abingdon
Oxon OX14 1AA
United Kingdom

www.radcliffepublishing.com

Electronic catalogue and worldwide online ordering facility.

British Library Cataloguing in Publication Data

A catalogue record for this book is available from the British Library.

ISBN-13: 978 184619 237 1

Typeset by Pindar NZ, Auckland, New Zealand
Printed and bound by Cadmus Communications, USA

Contents

Foreword

Choice is a word used daily in midwifery practice; it is supported through government documentations and has become part of every midwife's vocabulary. But choice is complex and is influenced by a number of complementary and competing factors. As a consequence, many researchers, including myself, have debated its contribution within maternity care. The breadth and depth of Julie's clinical and research experience has enabled her to capture the competing discourses in maternity care, providing real-life exemplars of the multidimensional nature of choice and its impact on care provision.

If one explores the many definitions of choice, four main attributes are identified. First, choice is a process, something that is negotiated internally and externally. Second, it relates to power and options; it is about having the right to choose, or not to. Third, it is about having more than one option; one cannot choose if there is nothing to choose between. Finally, it is about preference, and these are based on one's own personal values. This book captures all these elements in a comprehensive and thought-provoking way. It also demonstrates the process of knowledge acquisition, the relationship that this has with control and the resulting impact on maternity experiences and available services.

The implementation of 'choice' and enablement of 'control' relies on a complex interplay of individual and societal factors. This is beautifully illustrated throughout the book, as the author takes the reader on a journey which parallels that of women accessing maternity services. Julie provides a clear, comprehensive and well-referenced exposition throughout, presenting women's narratives in a powerful and dynamic way. This book demonstrates the value of storytelling as a valid research approach, and as a means of allowing practitioners to critique their own practice.

Maternal choice and control are a challenge in contemporary society, with the changing demography of the population, the rising birth rate and financial constraints. Collecting this diverse information in one publication is timely and an invaluable resource for the practising and academically active midwives, obstetricians and health service managers.

Tina Lavender
Professor of Midwifery
University of Manchester
August 2010

About the author

Julie Jomeen is a qualified nurse and midwife, who has worked at all clinical levels and also in a practice development role within a women and children's health department of a large acute trust. She is currently working as a Senior Lecturer in Midwifery and is Associate Dean, Research and Scholarship at the University of Hull, UK. Julie is involved in both pre- and post-registration teaching and postgraduate research supervision. Her research interests focus on issues around women's health and maternity care with a particular interest in psychological/mental health across the maternity spectrum and choice in healthcare, evidenced by numerous national and international publications and conference presentations.

Acknowledgements

There are some key people who deserve acknowledgement for their role in the writing of this book. The most enormous debt of gratitude must go to Professor Nancy Harding for her inspiration, encouragement and guidance for this work. Also special thanks must go to Professor Colin Martin, for his consistent support of my research endeavours and in particular for his guidance in the quantitative element of this study.

I must acknowledge my friends and colleagues working within maternity services who allowed me to hijack their clinics to recruit women to the study. Particular and special thanks must go to Janet Cairns for her constant support and listening ear.

A big thank you to Omar, Ellie and Aaron for their unfailing tolerance, love and support.

Thanks must also go to the Economic and Social Research Council for providing the funding that enabled this project to happen.

Last, but certainly not least, I want to firstly thank the women who gave their time to take part in this study and huge thanks in particular to those women who shared with me their stories so openly, honestly and willingly. Without them this book would not have been possible.

Introduction

Current policy advocates choice and control for women within maternity care and promotes women as active childbirth consumers and decision-makers.[1,2] This model equates choice to increased quality of experience and improved emotional outcomes, in the recognition that pregnancy and childbirth are both physical and psychological experiences. This is a response to the critique of the traditional biomedical model of pregnancy, which prioritises the physical aspects of pregnancy and advocates monitoring and surveillance to ensure fetal well-being. However, what informed choice means and whether it is desirable or possible remains central to debates within maternity care,[3] with the concept of choice contained within contemporary policy remaining questionable. For example, the assumption of a sharp distinction between the physiological and the psychological is not so straightforward and the ongoing tension between these two stances may leave women caught in the middle as both consumers and recipients of care. Further, choice is a desire but also a rational act, intimate connections between reason and rationality require a weighing up of risks and benefits and an ordering of preferences based on their utility.[4] Choice within such a frame would seem less straightforward than policy assumes. It appears to require women to balance their desire for a fulfilling birth experience with reasoned and rational decisions about their experience as a whole. Outcomes during pregnancy and birth are uncertain, so choice may not involve merely desire but also a gamble. Whilst in the developed world women can feel reassured that they are less likely than ever to die in pregnancy or childbirth, the growth of technology has brought new challenges to the pregnancy and birth experience. Medical experts hold perceptions of risk and in this sense have mapped out what women's 'responsible' decisions should be, to question or pay no attention to medicalised definitions of risk is to be seen as immoral or labelled a 'bad mother'.[5]

Policy makers in responding to public critiques of the biomedical model, have led us to believe that choice and control are always both desired and possible for women accessing maternity care.[6] In 2003, a decade after the influential document for maternity services, Changing Childbirth, had first introduced the concepts of choice and control, a House of Commons Health Committee report on maternity services was still questioning maternity choice as 'an illusion' and urging the Department of Health to ensure women received genuine and informed choice. It seems that little in this regard has changed, with a number of authors continuing to highlight barriers to choice and questioning its authenticity.[7,8,9] Moreover, robust evidence of the improvement in psychological outcomes that might have been expected as a result of choice of maternity care, has also failed to transpire.[10,11] Despite the official focus upon woman-centred childbirth and a move to encourage women to make decisions about their care in both physical and social terms, there remains a lack of consistent evidence with regard to expected benefits or the 'reality of choice' for women making choices for the management of childbirth. Indeed, the model of choice presupposes that pregnant women are a homogeneous category. This remains ignorant of the individual, complex and multidimensional nature of women's experiences of childbirth. Pregnant women's voices generally remain somewhat silent in the debates surrounding choice, and to inform the discussions and practices about choice, exploration of their 'reality' is the only real way to understand whether choice is discernable and significant in women's childbirth experiences.

WOMEN'S LIVED PREGNANCY AND CHILDBIRTH EXPERIENCES

Pregnancy and birth is a profound event in women's lives and how it is experienced has significant and enduring meaning for those women. This book presents some experiences of women who took part in a research study that set out to investigate and explore women's experiences of maternity care choice. It is important to acknowledge early in this book that the findings presented here were produced as part of a larger mixed-methods study exploring the 'Impact of Choice of Care on Antenatal and Postnatal Psychological Health Outcomes'. Whilst the results of the quantitative aspect of the study are relevant and will be referred to within this book, they have been primarily reported elsewhere,[10] the purpose of this book is rather to share women's lived experiences through stories they told as part of the study. Whilst I make no apologies for utilising such a methodological approach, many others would argue that methodological eclecticism is philosophically and politically incoherent, and so it feels necessary to provide some context through the methodological journey of this study. Denis Walsh suggests that models of midwifery care fall into the category of complex interventions and that quantitative methods alone, have a limited usefulness when evaluating all the distinctions of continuity of care, midwifery-led care, case load models and birth-centre care.[11] Informed by feminist perspectives, an underpinning premise for the methodological decision-making of this study was to acknowledge, utilise and counter the critique that using a quantitative approach to knowledge generation about choice would continue to situate women's experience within the bio-medical cause and effect frame.

As individuals we hold a set of beliefs about the world, which can be described as our personal paradigms. A paradigm is a conceptual framework on or around which we can create and construct our ideas about knowledge. It is generally believed that researchers' ontological and epistemological beliefs, that is how one firstly understands the nature of reality and then on which basis knowledge claims can be made, will lead to the resultant personal paradigm in which an individual situates themselves. This will in turn influence and guide methodological choices and actions during the research process,[13] and dictate the research strategy, methodology and method adopted. It can be argued, however, that knowledge should be evaluated in terms of how it should guide actions towards the realisation of particular objectives, which are the expressions of particular needs or interests, that in turn require reflection from the researcher upon the nature of the research with regard to human consequences.[14] It was a belief within this work that midwifery is a combination of the natural and the social sciences,[15] and that pregnancy and childbirth, as experiences that exist on more than one level, are more than one single reality and hence require more than one way of being understood. Midwifery research has been critiqued for traditionally adopting masculine models of knowing and midwives for being agents of the medical model.[16] This definition of masculine knowing must imply feminine models of knowing and female ways of accessing it, which would seem more consistent with the concept of the midwife being 'with woman'. However, there is no consistent feminist orthodoxy and there are many different feminisms, what these different approaches and I share is a common agreement about the centrality of the critical analysis of relationships in research and theory, an appreciation that women are worthy of study in their own right and the recognition of the need for social change to improve the lives of women.[17] Central, therefore to the values of this research was how to promote feminine ways of knowing when masculine ways of knowing traditionally dominate, it was thus incongruous to present a theory of the impact of choice of care on women's maternity experience based purely on a discourse presented through a quantitative predominantly male lens. There are those who believe that objective scientific approach is the only sound basis for knowledge production and hence subjective knowledge is unreliable. There are others who believe that qualitative methods are the only way of allowing a grasp of women's realities. However, any methodology can be considered feminist if women's voices are prioritised.[18] Two key concepts appear to prevail within feminist approaches, empowerment of women and equality of the research relationship. A clear priority for this research was to ensure outcomes that would contribute and impact on women's care provision and health in pregnancy, childbirth and beyond, and that any knowledge claims would be embedded in women's realities.

THE STUDY

The women involved in this study had already consented to and been involved in the quantitative aspect of the study. The women for the larger quantitative study had been sampled according to maternal choice of maternity care, which included:

➤ consultant-led care with intended birth at a large city maternity unit
➤ midwifery-led care with intended birth at a large city maternity unit
➤ midwifery-led care with intended birth at a stand-alone birth centre.

It should be noted here that it would also have been ideal to include a home birth group in the study, but the unfortunate fact that the number of home births within the locality was so small at the time that it was unfeasible to do so, speaks for itself. Ten women self-selected to take part in the qualitative aspect of the study, and it must be acknowledged that as a result the sample of women was probably predisposed to perceive the subject as important. Recruitment took place in 2003 and I followed these women across the period of a year, interviewing them twice during the antenatal period (10–14 weeks pregnant and 32 weeks pregnant) and twice during the postnatal period (14 days postnatal and 6 months postnatal).

Amongst the 10 women interviewed, there were representatives from within all three defined care groups. All the participants were white and originated from two geographical areas in the North of England but were demographically quite diverse. Five women were having their first baby and the remaining five were having their second or third babies. The women who already had children previously had a traditional model of care and hospital births. One woman previously had a caesarean section, the others had birthed normally. In relation to the labour and birth women experienced whilst taking part in this study, I will let the women tell their own stories. The views of the 10 women who took part in this study cannot be said to be necessarily representative of the wider population but this was not the purpose of this aspect of the research. The stories women shared rather allowed interpretations and theories to develop around women's maternity experiences. Whilst the central tenet of this research was women's experiences of choice in maternity care, in reality women told much broader stories. Women often referred to their previous birth experiences to explain and explore their feelings during their current experience and they were encouraged to do so. The belief was that the articulation of their previous experience enabled them to make sense of their current birth, labour and postnatal experience.

The interviews with the women were designed as conversational in approach and as a result lasted between an hour and three hours. Feminist researchers stress 'the importance of achieving symmetry in the social identities of the interview pair'[19] and it was important in this study that women were not utilised merely as sources of data. Women were giving a great deal in terms of their time and access to their intimate thoughts and feelings at this time in their lives therefore, some personal investment in the research relationship seemed imperative. Oakley states that finding out about people is best achieved in a non-hierarchical relationship between the interviewee and the interviewer, and benefits from an investment by the researcher of his or her personal identity.[20]

My aim throughout the interviews was to enable women to tell their birth stories. In order to promote women's voices, understanding how they made sense of their experience was crucial and in order to do that I have tried to be faithful to women's accounts. The stories that women tell challenge the doctrine about choice in maternity care. It should be explicitly expressed that throughout this book pregnancy and birth are recognised as being surrounded by complex social processes. Developing an understanding of women's maternity experiences necessitates a need to go beyond the traditional biological, psychological and sometimes superficial social accounts that characterise the literature. It is important to assess how women respond to pregnancy and how policies such as choice impact. However, there is a further need to comprehend the meanings and understanding that women attach to the emotional experiences of being pregnant, giving birth and adapting to life after the birth of their babies.

How childbirth and life interact is multifaceted and having a baby does not exist in a biological vacuum, but within a social, historical and political context, which inevitably must shape and influence how women experience all aspects of pregnancy and birth. The findings presented in this book are based on the belief that the social world in which the women are living, is powerfully constructed by human beliefs and attitudes about roles and identities, which in turn shape practices, behaviours and in the case of this particular research, choices and psychological health. Thus in this context, women's realities are regarded as multidimensional. The social experiences of these women can be best understood through subjective interpretation and mental constructions; this is not to claim that the experiences they display through more objective measures are imaginary. However, the beliefs that underpin this work acknowledge that there are multiple realities and that individuals understand their socially constructed reality through lived experience and competing human perceptions of the truth (if such a thing exists), constructed out of what people recognise as facts.[21]

The research within this book is significantly influenced by feminist theory, but also theoretically driven by the literature on the psychology and sociology of childbirth, both the institution and ideologies of motherhood, and the discourses surrounding maternity care. The narratives constructed through the interviews with women will undoubtedly reflect those discourses, as they are influential in my own consciousness and experience, and inevitably influence my interpretation of the stories told.

THE VALUE OF STORYTELLING TO UNDERSTANDING WOMEN'S MATERNITY EXPERIENCES

Narrative and stories are fundamental ways of giving meaning to experience. Most stories concern social interaction and concern events as experienced by specific actors. Telling stories allows narrators to communicate what is significant in their lives and how things matter to them.[22] Narratives have a primary function that involves bringing order to disorder; in telling a story the narrator is trying to organise the disorganised into some form of meaning,[23] and narrative mediates between an inner world of thought and feeling and an outer world of states of affairs.[22] Tension can then exist for narrators in trying to give meaning to the various challenges and disruptions to the order of everyday life. Pregnancy can be perceived as such a disruption and a challenge to women and narrative provides a primary means of restoring such order. Therefore stories can provide a powerful medium for learning and gaining understanding about others, by affording a context for insights into personal experiences. They can promote understandings of social, cultural and moral orders, and offer a way of constructing reality that deals in purpose and action and the change of state and consequences that mark their path.[24]

The meaning that the women interviewed attribute to childbirth, reflects their expectations and understandings gained through participating in a specific social and moral world of pregnancy and motherhood. Humans are hubs of action who strive within their own to create their worlds.[23] As a consequence women narrated experiences that implied their role or lack of it in shaping events. Paul Ricoeur[23] developed an immense body of work on the centrality of narrative for meaning making, and argues that individuals need to create narratives to bring order and meaning, but further that narrative is central to how we conceive of ourselves, to our very identity and self definition. It is through narrative that we construct connectedness to others but it is also how we distinguish ourselves from others.[23] The interactions with the women, in this study, aimed to promote a better understanding of the emotional, cultural and social grounding of their experiences through the stories constructed. Narratives, unlike discourses, have a finished structure, although the full dimensions of the structure require the reader to complete the narrative.[23] It is this completion that draws on the established social narratives within which both teller and audience live. Hence, it is necessary to acknowledge that narrative is open to alternative readings as it deals with human possibilities not fixed beliefs.[24] It is also important to note that all narratives are provisional, they are subject to change as new information becomes available. Women in their early pregnancy narratives were not aware of the outcomes of their pregnancies, their birth experiences or their adaptation to motherhood but could only relate their worlds and identities as they saw them at that point in time or in the context of expected outcomes. Hollway and Jefferson suggest that the form of a person's account is the sum of all the links that have been made within the available material,[19] and these women's narratives could not be complete until the final interview and only complete as far as this study was concerned. That is why in order to understand how women really encountered choice throughout their childbirth experience, it felt important to present the women's stories in full across their experience rather than dissect it into its different temporal components

The possibility of narrative discourse within this study was a way to bring women and their particular experiences of pregnancy, childbirth and motherhood into focus alongside the recognition that there is more to the story of being a 'maternity patient' than can be captured by a medical synopsis or objective measurement. Hence narrative provides an opportunity to distinguish childbirth as a phenomenon seen from a practitioner and professional's perspective, from childbirth as phenomena seen from the perspective of the women who experience it.

INTERVIEWING THE WOMEN AND THE RESEARCH RELATIONSHIP

Women's research is often characterised by an approach that sees the subjectivity of both researcher and subjects studied as central, in the first case through empathy and commitment, and in the second through personal experience. A mutual relationship of trust is essential, for without it we cannot be confident that our research on women's lives actually represents what is significant to them about their experience. Furthermore it assists in the acquisition of significant and meaningful data.[20] A feminist interviewer is by definition both part of and participating in the culture that she seeks to observe,[25] which involve the political considerations that flow from the researcher's own identity. Narratives resulting from interview are always a product of the relationship between the interviewer and interviewee. The work of Ann Oakley[20, 25] was the key to how I approached the interviews with the women in this study.

Oakley relates her experience of interviewing women in a research project concerned with the transition to motherhood. In her study she considers she was present during a critical phase in women's lives.[25] Oakley interviewed the women twice during pregnancy and twice after the birth of their babies, much the same as this study. She cites the difficulties that she encountered as twofold. Firstly the number of questions the women asked her and secondly that repeated interviewing which by its nature of involving women's intensely personal experiences of pregnancy, birth and motherhood established a basis of personal involvement that defies the representation of the proper interview as defined within a scientific frame.[25] Oakley further suggests that avoiding this personal involvement is ultimately unhelpful. Interviewing in the literature is often presented as a 'one-off' affair, where detachment is easier to maintain than in a longer-term research relationship. The women in this study volunteered for interview, so it would be expected that they wanted to talk about their experiences, however, similar to Oakley's experience they were also interested in my own situation. In addition they also often set the scene for the interview relationship as something beyond questions and answers and welcomed me into their homes offering drinks and even on occasions lunch. Declaration of my status as a mother within these interviews appeared to be regarded as a position of empathy, understanding and equality with the women's own experiences. Oakley, comments that where both interviewer and interviewee share the same gender, socialisation and critical life experiences, social distance can be minimal.[20] All questions about personal experience of pregnancy, birth and motherhood were answered honestly, although always from a positive perspective. My role as a midwife was integral in gaining access to these women as participants in the research. However that status was deliberately underplayed throughout, with the aim of minimising the power relations implicit in any interview situation. Women did, however, take the opportunity to ask for clinical advice, and as with the personal questions, I had made a conscious decision that I would answer these questions, which I did so as fully as I could without access to the case notes. I stressed that these were generic answers based on my midwifery experience not necessarily based on the interviewees' own situation. These approaches overall seemed to foster a feeling of intimacy and trust and seemed to aid and not hinder the informal atmosphere of the interviews. Women seemed to feel equally able to narrate negative as well as positive experiences with regard to midwives and their care generally, which suggests that my professional role, although it undoubtedly impacted on the interview relationship, did not discourage them from narrating their relevant stories.

In the case of these interviews, some were more difficult than others and some women were undoubtedly easier to relate to than others and it is relevant to consider how the women themselves must have perceived me. Although my aim was to dispense with the traditional power status normally adopted during research interviews, it of course should be acknowledged that my presence as a researcher, the environment and the cultural context would all continue to have influence. Despite my attempts above to minimise the power relations in the interview, some interviews required much more prompting and intervention in order to encourage response, and also to develop a sense early on that what these women had to say was actually of importance and value. This seemed to have the desired effect as even the more difficult interview relationships seemed to evolve over time and exchanges became more fluent and storied in their content. Women felt able to challenge the points I was making and take more control of the interview. The importance for me was in the privileging of women's experiences and treating all those experiences as equally valid. In narrative the agenda must be left open to change and development and adopting this approach did allow women the opportunity to talk freely about their experiences. Story telling can be differentiated from the products of traditional research interview by the narrator's own role in taking responsibility for making the relevance of the story clear.[19]

At times this obviously required digression from the traditional interviewing approach of asking the question and then engaging in good listening. This approach has also been criticised for its over confidence in the existence of true or genuine experiences and in the possibility of capturing these and it must be acknowledged that by asking questions we produce answers only through one frame, and no frame is ever neutral. However, Hollway and Jefferson firmly contend that the researchers interventions can be positive and instrumental in promoting mutual understanding and enhancing trust, and, are ultimately beneficial rather than exploitative for the interviewee.[19]

OVERVIEW OF CHAPTERS

The purpose of this book is to explore the experiences of women within contemporary maternity care and to understand their situation with particular reference to choice and control. The introduction has aimed to establish the orientation of the book and provide the context within which women's experiences will be explored and presented. Part 1 consists of Chapters 1 to 3.

Chapter 1 provides an overview and critical guide to current maternity policy and contemporary political rhetoric, with a particular emphasis on the concepts of choice and control. Chapter 2 provides an overview of the competing discourses of maternity care, which both women and maternity care providers are subjected to. Chapter 3 presents and briefly reviews some of the literature, theories and debates surrounding mothering and motherhood, and proposes a type of mothering that begins much earlier than the birth of the baby. Part 2 will then present and analyse the experiences of women who were interviewed across their maternity experience. The narratives that were produced explore women's experiences as pregnant women, women giving birth and new mothers. Chapter 4 reflexively outlines the development of the analytical framework that underpinned the qualitative data exploration and interpretation, which is unique to this study and based on a synthesis of narrative and semiotic models. Whilst this chapter may seem somewhat theoretical it feels essential to be transparent about how the interpretations presented in the subsequent chapters were reached. Chapters 5 to 8 utilise the analytical model developed to explore the influences and discourses revealed in women's antenatal and postnatal narratives and the resultant multiple identities created for women, within the context of maternity choices. Chapter 9 is the concluding section of this book and offers some overall thoughts, with regard to choice, interwoven with some recommendations for maternity service delivery and practice, as well as some future research recommendations.

REFERENCES

1 Department of Health, Department of Education and Skills. *National Service Framework for Children, Young People and Maternity Services: Maternity Services*. London: Department of Health; 2004.

2 Department of Health. *Maternity Matters: choice, access and continuity of care in a safe service*. London: Department of Health; 2007.

3 Kirkham M. *Informed Choice in Maternity Care*. Basingstoke: Palgrave Macmillan; 2004.

4 Allingham M. *Choice Theory: a very short introduction*. New York: Oxford University Press; 2002.

5 Edwards NP, Murphy-Lawless J. The instability of risk: womens' perspectives on risk and safety in birth. In: Symon A, editor. *Risk and Choice in Maternity Care: an international perspective*. Philadelphia: Churchill Livingstone; 2006.

6 Hunt S, Symonds A. *The Social Meaning of Midwifery*. Basingstoke: Macmillan Press; 1995.

7 Hollins-Martin CJ. How can we improve choice provision for childbearing women? *Br J Midwifery*. 2007; **15**(8): 480–4.

8 Jomeen J. Choice in Childbirth: a realistic expectation? *Br J Midwifery*. 2007; **15**(8): 485–90.

 9 Kightley R. Delivering choice: where to birth? *Br J Midwifery*. 2007; **15**(8): 475–8.

10 Jomeen J, Martin CR. The impact of choice of maternity care on psychological health outcomes for women during pregnancy and the postnatal period. *J Eval Clin Pract*. 2008; **14**(3): 391–8.

11 Renfrew MJ, Green JM, Spiby H. *Evidence submitted to the House of Commons Health Committee Maternity Sub-committee 1st inquiry (2003:03)*. Mother and Infant Research Unit: University of Leeds.

12 Walsh D. *Evidence-based Care for Normal Labour and Birth: a guide for midwives*. Abingdon: Routledge; 2007.

13 Norton L. The philosophical bases of grounded theory and their implications for research practice. *Nurse Res*. 1999; **7**(1): 31–43.

14 Gill J, Johnson P. *Research Methods for Managers*. 3rd ed. London: Sage; 2002.

15 Donovan P. Alternative approaches to research. In: Cluett ER, Bluff R, editors. *Principles and Practices of Research in Midwifery*. Edinburgh: Balliere Tindall; 2000.

16 Cluett ER, Bluff R, editors. *Principles and Practices of Research in Midwifery*. Edinburgh: Balliere Tindall; 2000.

17 Ussher JM. Feminist approaches to qualitative health research. In: Murray M, Chamberlain K, editors. *Qualitative Health Psychology: theories and methods*. London: Sage; 1999.

18 Millen D. Some methodological and epistemological issues raised by doing feminist research on non-feminist women. *Socio Res*. 1997; **2**(3): 1–34.

19 Hollway W, Jefferson T. *Doing Qualitative Research Differently*. 3rd ed. London: Sage; 2000.

20 Oakley A. Interviewing women: a contradiction in terms. In: Roberts H, editor. *Doing Feminist Research*. London: Routledge; 1981.

21 Gatrell C. *Hard Labour: the sociology of parenthood*. Maidenhead: Open University Press; 2005.

22 Mattingley C, Garro L. *Narrative and the Cultural Construction of Illness and Healing*. London: University of California Press; 2000.

23 Murray M. Narrative psychology. In: Smith JA, editor. *Qualitative Psychology*. London: Sage; 2003.

24 Bruner J. *Actual Minds, Possible Worlds*. Cambridge: Harvard University Press; 1986.

25 Oakley A. *The Ann Oakley Reader: gender, women and social science*. Bristol: Policy Press; 2005.

PART 1

Policy, theories and perspectives

CHAPTER 1

The context of choice in pregnancy and childbirth

The dominant medical philosophy of management of women in pregnancy is that pregnancy is a condition that can only be considered normal in retrospect and in labour is primarily focussed on the efficient and safe removal of the fetus from the mother.[1] In this context problems are not only solved but defined by experts with specialist knowledge, with the experts traditionally being medical practitioners.[2] This medicalised and risk averse approach has resulted in a high value been placed on detection of abnormality, defining all women, not just those with potential complications, as needing hospitalisation and medical surveillance and input. However, such a framework also resulted in a workforce of medicalised midwives.[3] Despite more recent and innovative changes in the way midwives deliver care to pregnant women, many midwives continue to work in obstetric technology driven units, creating an obstetric ideology that Nadine Edwards refers to as coercive, suggesting that while minor choices exist, conceptual choices do not.[4] It is unsurprising in such a context that issues surrounding women's personal control and choice in a childbirth context were, until relatively recently, viewed as of secondary concern and a labouring woman's perspective was often not acknowledged during childbirth by the clinical staff determining her care.[5]

THE POLICY CONTEXT

Improving the experience of childbirth for women was nationally prioritised through Changing Childbirth,[6] the report prioritised individuality of women's needs, their need for information, involvement in planning care, an ongoing relationship with a lead professional and accessibility of services. The three central tenets of that document were choice, control and continuity. Changing

Childbirth was a product of the wider strategic healthcare reforms of the 1980s and 1990s, a politically determined attempt to make healthcare services more market orientated and consumer driven. The document emerged directly from the House of Commons Health Select Committee Maternity Report,[7] which had concluded that maternity care should no longer be driven by a medical model of care. The Changing Childbirth document clearly reflected the views of consumers as well as professionals. The aims of the document were to be achieved within a bold five-year timescale, and a number of pilot schemes emerged in an attempt to meet the policy doctrine. However, despite success in meeting their intended aims very few of these schemes were enduring in nature, in a large part linked to cost and a failure to find recurring funding, leaving both consumers and midwives disheartened and cynical. The Changing Childbirth document was however a seminal one and the forerunner of subsequent and current policy. Whilst policy language has evolved since the early 1990s, continuity appears to have become 'women-centred care' and new words such as 'flexible' and 'accessible' have entered the rhetorical arena, choice remains a popular word within political vocabulary. Documents such as the National Service Framework, Maternity Standard 11[8] and Maternity Matters[9] lucidly illustrated choice as an integral part of contemporary maternity care. Maternity Matters stressed 'a wider choice in maternity care' and laid down choice guarantees (p. 5), which included choice of how to access maternity care, type of antenatal care, place of birth and postnatal care. Unlike its predecessor Changing Childbirth, the implementation of Maternity Matters was accompanied by a monitoring framework, which was included in the document.[9] However, recent healthcare reports and reviews[10] suggest that many trusts are falling well short of these targets.

Maternity policy under a labour government has reflected wider government policy in relation to a contemporary NHS, including the recent Darzi report.[11] Although Darzi said little about maternity care in particular, it did comment on the need for a more personalised NHS, responsive to each of us as individuals, giving us real choices over our care and our lives, commenting specifically that women want greater choice over place of birth.[11] Despite a change of government, the most recent publication 'Liberating the NHS', sees the rhetoric of choice for women within maternity services persist, with the continued recognition that any choice offered needs to be informed and safe (p.17).[12]

WOMEN AND CHOICE

As evidence for some time has pointed out, women themselves appear to desire choice in maternity care.[13] Women state that they would prefer more choice about the type of care and site for delivery.[11] A postal survey identified that a large minority of women (46%) when assessed antenatally and postnatally did not feel that they had exercised informed choice overall in their maternity care. Of particular interest is that informed choice differed by decision point and whilst it was reported as high for decisions such as screening for Down's syndrome and spina bifida it was low for interventions such as fetal monitoring in labour, which are more likely to be determined by professional perceptions of risk.[14]

Choice implies both knowledge and understanding, and assumes that individuals make choices based on wants or needs and the ability to assess and dismiss alternatives. It is suitably acknowledged that choice is not an equitable concept, low income, poor housing and nutrition are all inequalities recognised to restrict access to services, increase risk[8,9] and consequently decrease choice.[15] Kightley highlights the increase in female headed lone-parent households and suggests that in such households the choice of a hospital delivery may be a choice for support, that a woman might not otherwise have access to because of her single status, rather than a choice for the type of birth experience she would prefer.[16] It is important to recognise that women make choices for a whole set of often complex reasons and it should not be assumed that the decision to have a hospital birth is the wrong one.[16] However, we also know that choice is constructed through pervading belief systems and resources[4] and the recent Birth Place Choices study demonstrated that the majority of women, continue to cite hospital 'as the best place to give birth' and make choices according to the continued social construction of hospital as the safest place for birth.[17] Kightley further suggests that in the UK, hospital birth can be seen as the birthing tradition of many indigenous women of childbearing age, a legacy from their mothers who were told and believed that hospital was the safest place for them and their babies.[16] This potentially creates tensions for women between a desired birth experience and the need to be seen to make responsible and safe choices. Safety is a key issue in maternity care and despite the fact that childbirth has never been safer, in terms of mortality, fear of birth amongst mothers remains,[18] recently highlighted by the new diagnostic category of tokophobia (morbid fear of labour). Fear is also an influential factor in terms of the professional culture surrounding maternity care[19] and relevant here is the risk discourse surrounding pregnancy, which will be discussed in more detail in Chapter 2.

MIDWIVES AND CHOICE

The Royal College of Midwives has consistently supported client choice with regard to the place of birth, and encourages midwives to offer choice.[16] Studies demonstrate, however, that midwives restrict information to certain groups of women, depending on risk assessment and their own personal experiences.[17]

Edwards suggests that there are differences between midwives individual ideologies and the ideology of the system within which they practise.[4] Such findings ask fundamental questions of the Maternity Matters choice guarantees. The document itself states that 'Choice is dependent on circumstances' and 'for some women, team care will be the safest option'.[9] Within such a model, options and choices for those women identified as 'high risk' are immediately constrained and a desired pregnancy and birth experience becomes secondary to perceptions of risk and concerns about safety.

A choice framework assumes a democratic model, where the woman is expected to be able to exercise her rights and make choices.[3] However, much of the information is held and its nature determined by healthcare professionals, as such decisions are not made from a level playing field.[15] Women are entitled to make informed choices about any aspect of their maternity experience they want regarding place of birth, type of birth, pain relief in labour and method of feeding, to name a few, as long as it is the choice we, as professionals, think they should make. A system of rights based on guilt and blame is unlikely to create a context in which women can assert their own knowledge, desires and need. Examples exist of women's negative experiences when they have declined professional advice and made a choice for an unadvised course of action.

> [A]nd I said look at the end of the day it's my right to choose a home confinement . . . this is what I want and this is what I'm happy with. And she said well I don't think I can support you in this decision. In my opinion I think you're making the wrong choice. I don't think home is the right place for you to have your first child. You don't know what its going to be like. You don't know what complications you are going to have and goodness knows anything could go wrong and you know you could end up putting yourself and your child in danger. Do you want your unborn child to die? . . . It left me feeling very isolated . . . you end up with self-doubt – whether you are making the right decision or whether you are strong enough to actually go the whole way with it (p. 16).[4]

Very few women, of course, go against professional advice; most women will not make choices that they perceive might alienate those providing them with care. The Royal College of Midwives , comments that women tend toward compliance when they perceive that they or more especially their baby is at risk.[20] Studies have demonstrated that experts in the form of medical and midwifery personnel continue to be viewed by women as knowing best and as such play a vital role in constraining or facilitating women's choice. The gatekeeping role played by some GPs in both facilitating and impeding choice has been demonstrated, and whilst women who experienced barriers to choice expressed discontent, the

GP remained fundamentally unchallenged.[21] Midwives have also been accused of being complicit in ways of working and advising that incorporate a medical model.[3] Weaver demonstrated how midwives through their own personal opinions represent home birth as hazardous to women, which in turn leads women to express similar fears.[22] The legacy of the medical model, with depictions of pregnancy and birth as a risky process, continues to emphasise hospital and expert intervention as the means to assure the safety of the baby, which constrains women's choices through fear.[21]

Guideline-driven care standardises clinical behaviour, and further reinforces a right course of action or choice particularly when deviation from the pathway requires written justification.[23] Such an approach fails to support midwives autonomy and in turn compromises the midwives ability to facilitate women's autonomy. Risk protocols and evidence based care are seemingly often incompatible with choice. Hollins-Martin and Bull further demonstrated how midwives feel obliged to obey a senior midwife and when conflicts arise the obedience to the senior person is prioritised over being an advocate for a women's choice.[24,25] Many midwives experienced impediments to their ability to provide and support women's choice. These included hospital policies, hierarchical control and fearing consequences of challenging senior staff, which in turn comprised of fear of an abnormal obstetric outcome, litigation, conflict and intimidation.[25] It should be acknowledged that senior staff are also part of a hierarchy and within that hierarchy are expected to implement standardised procedures and guidelines. In this position they may also find supporting choice difficult.[26]

It is important to emphasise that whilst it is well documented that midwives can constrain women's choices through their attitudes, beliefs and the inherent power balance in the relationship, many midwives actively seek to support women's choices despite difficult circumstances and often being uncertain about outcomes themselves.[27]

BENEFITS OF CHOICE

Limited research evidence has evaluated the benefits of choice for women in maternity care. Maternity care choices have been linked to maternal satisfaction[28,29] and personal control.[18,30] One framework through which the benefits and detriments of choice have been discussed is autonomy, and Nadine Edwards claims that decreasing autonomy risks decreasing women's sense of self-worth, self-trust, self esteem and confidence, and further may undermine the self.[4] This suggests that when women are enabled to be autonomous that there are significant associated psychological benefits. However, the choice of maternity care, as a single independent variable does not, it seem, lead to the psychological benefits expected.[31,32] Indeed, findings suggested that women experience similar physical and psychological challenges across the maternity spectrum, regardless of the choices they make for care.[31] One of the key difficulties is that woman make choices for maternity care with no real knowledge of what is ahead in pregnancy and choices made can become impossible to fulfil if the 'risk status' of the pregnancy changes and decision-making regarding the pregnancy and or birth then inevitably becomes remit of the experts rather than the woman.[21] Further explanations for a lack of empirical evidence to support the psychological benefits of choice are that choice is simply not a reality for women, it is an illusory concept with lip service featuring prominently,[33] and more likely rhetorical to the point of non-existence.[34] The limiting of women's autonomy and the controlling of choices by practitioners makes it impossible for a woman to make true choices,[34,35] making associations between choice and outcomes impossible to determine. Whilst such claims seem to provide an intuitive interpretation of the quantitative element of our study, it is also possible to propose that women across the groups were satisfied with the choices made and so choice had indeed led to psychological benefits. Such an interpretation, however, is undermined by the psychological profiles displayed by women across the groups. All women worried about socio-medical aspects of pregnancy with worries highest in late pregnancy, further the findings in relation to control suggested that in pregnancy women believe that 'powerful others' (which would include the midwife as well as the doctor) have control over events governing their health but more illuminating is that this increased external control appears to compromise women's internal control.[31] This latter finding might make it feasible to suggest a further explanation, which is that the positive outcomes credited to choice are rather associated with issues of control. The issue of control will be discussed in more detail in the next section

Choice has been a policy theme notoriously hard to fulfil. Fifteen plus years on from Changing Childbirth, evidence suggests that fundamentally little has changed,[36] and the 'reality of choice' remains elusive despite the continuing official focus.

CHOICE AND CONTROL

Shelia Kitzinger acknowledges that 'the debate about control is challenging because there is little agreement about what the word means' (p. 12).[37]

Evidence seems to suggest that the constructs of choice and control are intimately connected for women with regard to pregnancy and their childbirth experience. The opportunity for greater choice over care allows more involvement with decision-making and impacts on a woman's feelings of control. In a study by Walker, women choosing delivery in a midwife-led unit formulated a very clear idea about the type of experience they wanted for the birth of their baby and loss of choice was found to be an important reason for feelings of loss of control.[38] In her study exploring women's experiences of home birth, Nadine Edwards illustrates how technology can cause women to feel a loss of control.[35]

> I did feel (in control) unless I was strapped onto the monitor and then it really changed me. So no, I didn't feel very much in control then but when I was doing all my different positions I was completely in control (p. 232).[35]

Gatrell's work with professional women demonstrated the physical and mental affects for women when they felt deprived of choice and information. Whilst women did not object to medical intervention per se all women found it difficult when it robbed them of a sense of control during pregnancy and birth. Also noteworthy in that same study were the, albeit small number of women (n=3) who reported depression for up to three years following a perceived traumatic birth, seemingly exacerbated by the feelings that they had lost any sense of control during pregnancy or birth.[39] These women suggested that loss of control had robbed them of self-confidence and self-esteem in all aspects of their lives for a considerable time. Such interpretations are consistent with Green, Coupland and Kitzinger,[18] who, in their large study examining the psychological effects of childbirth on mothers, found that the perception of feeling in control was reliably and consistently related to positive psychological outcomes. Other studies have concurred with these findings. Lavender, Walkinshaw and Walton revealed control to be amongst the themes contributing to women's views of a positive birth experience.[40] A study by Schneider using a qualitative framework found that control emerged as an important issue even in the first trimester.[41] Studies have identified that women seem to judge most situations by the degree of control they feel they can maintain.[42] Maushart, however, suggests that it is the illusion of control over their bodies that is important to women,[43] and Green and Baston propose that women are more concerned about negotiated levels of control and that any surrender of control is voluntary.[43] Women themselves are not always clear what they mean by control; control can relate to many aspects of pregnancy such as behaviour, decisions related to her pregnancy, control during labour and delivery, or control over the course and direction of her pregnancy. Women may demonstrate awareness of the changes that are happening in pregnancy, and feel conflict as a result of the difference between their self-perception of being in control and discomfort as a result of those things 'just happening to their bodies'.[41] This may leave women feeling a loss of control reinforced by their inability to relieve the physical symptoms of pregnancy, labour and birth.

Personal perceived control has been found to be an important determinant of women's satisfaction with their birth experience.[44] Personal control has been found to be dependent upon pregnant women having options that allowed choice, adequate information and involvement in the decision-making process. It is suggested that a midwife is the professional best placed to provide access to adequate information,[45] and so women receiving midwifery-led care might be expected to demonstrate greater levels of personal control. A study of women with negative memories of their first birth having a subsequent home birth, found that women felt able to exercise control over their subsequent deliveries due to the role of the caregiver, who enabled them to overcome personal characteristics including low self-esteem and obedience to authority.[46] However, Edwards exploring control in the context of women choosing and planning homebirths, found that whilst women initially felt that staying at home to give birth would enable them to remain in control, in reality they found the picture once again to be much more complex.[47] Whilst women could establish and maintain control over the environment, control and decision-making more broadly were dependant on similarity between midwives and women's views and beliefs, and the medicalised technocratic model often shaped information exchange and hence decision-making and control.[47] Edwards comments sadly that this reflects the findings reported over two decades earlier.

Choice and the notion of subsequent control are dependent on information gathering relevant to that woman's individual circumstances and entrusting her to make decisions. The rhetoric of choice and control offers a promise of autonomy for women but studies conducted using qualitative research methodologies have highlighted a loss of personal autonomy and control as a key theme for women during labour and childbirth.[35,48] Eakins, focusing on women who conceptualised childbirth as non-medical, found that they rejected the institutionalised hospital system in favour of attaining personal control; participants in postnatal interviews cited feeling in control as their most preferred aspect of the experience of labour and birth.[49] Cunningham found women choosing birth-centre and home births nominated the desire to have an active birth with control.[50] However, for some women control is conceptualised differently and may be linked to the 'safety net' of the hospital. In contrast to many other findings, a study investigating home versus hospital management of women with a pre-labour rupture of membranes, found women in the hospital group displayed higher internal locus of control (LOC) scores than those in the home group at the onset of labour or prior to induction of labour.[51] This suggests that those women in the hospital group actually felt more in control of events governing their health at that time. Whilst this may seem counter-intuitive in light of other evidence, one potential interpretation of these findings is that they reflect the medical and technocratic discourses that surround birth and with which women are presented. Brewin and Bradley investigating women's perceived control and the experience of childbirth did find that women who perceived themselves to be in control over their labour reported less pain, however, interestingly, less pain was also reported when they perceived the staff to have control over their labour.[52] Anderson suggests that the worst option for women seem to be when they believe that no-one has control over the labour and for labour to be 'out of control'.[53] Labour is inevitably a process where loss of control can occur and one solution to a feeling of loss of internal control is to seek external control. Gould suggests that when we believe things are out of our control we develop a fatalistic attitude.[54] This may proffer some explanation as to why generally women are overwhelmingly complicit with a handover of control during pregnancy and birth because to resist may compromise a safe outcome and the well-being of their baby.[21] What is clear is that the conceptualisation of control in pregnancy and childbirth is more complex than some of the literature has previously assumed, as is its relationship to choice.

More recent psychological studies have implicated the domain of personal control, in particular, low levels of perceived personal control, as being related to experience of post-traumatic stress symptoms following childbirth.[55] The authors suggest that developing care interventions that enhance perception of control has been suggested as a possible intervention to reduce the possibility of post-traumatic stress symptoms post-partum.[55] Scott-Palmer and Skevington found that women with an internal LOC orientation (women who felt more in control of events governing their health), had significantly shorter labours compared to women with an external LOC orientation (women who felt their health was governed either by chance or powerful others).[56] Tinsley and colleagues found that perceptions of personal control were associated with compliance to prenatal health regimes, which in turn were related strongly to actual birth outcomes.[57] This suggests that control during pregnancy and birth has far-reaching implications beyond those of satisfaction with care or experience.

The mother to be's perceived uniqueness of the experience of labour and childbirth has also been identified to influence LOC orientation. Lowe found that high levels of fear and apprehension regarding a forthcoming confinement were significantly associated with high levels of 'chance' and 'powerful others' health LOC.[58] Accumulating evidence seems to suggest that perceived control does interface with the psychobiological process of the woman's childbirth experience. As referred to above, the findings from the quantitative arm of this study[31] strengthen the claim that pregnancy per se compromises internal control. Pregnant women as a group demonstrated higher scores as measured by the Multidimensional Health Locus of Control Scale [MHLC[59]], 'others' (would include midwives), doctors and chance subscales, and lower scores on the internal subscale than non-pregnant counterparts. This suggests that women perceive internal control as compromised and their health as much more externally controlled, particularly in medical terms. This may not necessarily be a negative finding and other authors have demonstrated that control was rather related to how women perceived they were treated and consideration of caregivers was significantly and positively related to feelings of control.[30] The women's narratives presented later will provide a more nuanced perspective of the concept.

SUMMARY

It is acknowledged that childbirth represents a major transition in a woman's life and serves as a 'rite of passage' into the social institution of motherhood. Birthing is both a physical and psychological challenge and the manner in which a woman experiences birth is likely to affect her adjustment to motherhood.[60]

There is a clear and official focus and rhetoric of woman-centred childbirth, and choice and decisions about their care are an integral element of that rhetoric. Whilst policy changes imply a move away from a paternalistic and controlling model of childbirth to one that promotes autonomy, choice and control for women, robust evidence as to such a change and the tangible benefits of choice for women are lacking. Choices for some women are not a reality; other women may not always be clear about what it is they are choosing, and health professionals have been identified as often culpable in directing women's choices either through the information given or through not giving information at all.

Information-giving, choice, decision-making and control appear implicitly intertwined with a woman's pregnancy and birth experience, and increasingly compelling evidence suggests that it is an interaction between these variables that has significant implications for woman and their maternity experience. Women themselves, however, whilst desiring choice, are influenced by the powerful cultural discourses that surround maternity care. This will inevitably impact on the choice and decision they make.

REFERENCES

1 Rothman BK. Women, providers and control. *J Obstet Gynecol Neonatal Nurs.* 1996; 25: 253–6.

2 Gross H, Pattison H. *Sanctioning Pregnancy.* Hove: Routledge; 2007.

3 Kent J. *Social Perspectives on Pregnancy and Childbirth for Midwives, Nurses and the Caring Professions.* Buckingham: Open University Press; 2000.

4 Edwards NP. Why can't women just say no? And does it really matter? In: Kirkham M, editor. *Informed Choice in Maternity Care.* Basingstoke: Palgrave Macmillan; 2004.

5 Beaton JI. Dimension of nurse and patient roles in labour. *Health Care Women Int.* 1990; **11**: 393–408.

6 Department of Health. *Changing Childbirth.* London: HMSO; 1993.

7 House of Commons. *Health Committee Second Report. Session 1991–1992: Maternity Services.* London: HMSO; 1992.

8 Department of Health and Department of Education and Skills. *National Service Framework for Children, Young People and Maternity Services: Maternity Services.* London: Department of Health; 2004.

9 Department of Health. *Maternity Matters: choice, access and continuity of care in a safe service.* London: Department of Health; 2007.

10 Healthcare Commission. *Towards Better Births: a review of maternity services in England.* London: Healthcare Commission; 2008.

11 Department of Health. *High Quality Care for All: NHS Next Stage Review Final Report (Darzi).* London: Department of Health; 2008.

12 Department of Health. *Equity and Excellence: Liberating the NHS.* London: Department of Health; 2010.

13 Kirkham M. *Informed Choice in Maternity Care.* Basingstoke: Palgrave Macmillan; 2004.

14 O'Cathain A, Thomas K, Walters S, *et al.* Women's perceptions of informed choice in maternity care. *Midwifery.* 2002; **18**(2): 136–44.

15 Symon A. *Risk and Choice in Maternity Care: an international perspective.* Philadelphia: Churchill Livingstone; 2006.

16 Kightley R. Delivering choice: where to birth? *Br J Midwifery.* 2007; **15**(8): 475–8.

17 Barber T, Rogers J, Marsh S. Increasing out of hospital birth: what needs to change? *Br J Midwifery.* 2007; **15**(1): 16–20

18 Green JM, Coupland BA, Kitzinger J. Expectations, experiences and psychological outcomes of childbirth: a prospective study of 825 women. *Birth.* 1990; **17**: 15–24.

19 Kirkham M, Stapleton H. The culture of the maternity services in Wales and England as a barrier to informed choice. In: Kirkham M, editor. *Informed Choice in Maternity Care.* Basingstoke: Palgrave Macmillan; 2004.

20 Royal College of Midwives. *Reassessing Risk: a midwifery perspective.* London: Royal College of Midwives; 2000.

21 Jomeen J. Choice in childbirth: a realistic expectation? *Br J Midwifery.* 2007; **15**(8): 485–90.

22 Weaver J. Childbirth. In: Ussher JM, editor. *Women's Health: contemporary international perspectives.* Leicester: British Psychological Society; 2000.

23 Griffiths R. Maternity care pathways and the law. *Br J Midwifery.* 2009; **17**(4): 210.

24 Hollins-Martin CJ, Bull P. Measuring social influence of a senior midwife on decision-making in maternity care: an experimental study. *J Community Appl Soc.* 2005; **15**: 120–6.

25 Hollins-Martin CJ, Bull P. What features of the maternity unit promote obedient behaviour from midwives? *Clin Effect Nurs.* 2006; **952**: e221–31.

26 Hollins-Martin CJ. How can we improve choice provision for childbearing women? *Br J Midwifery.* 2007; **15**(8): 480–4.

27 Leap N. The less we do, the more we give. In: Kirkham M, editor. *The Midwife-Mother Relationship.* Basingstoke: Palgrave Macmillan; 2000.

28 Spurgeon P, Hicks C, Barwell F. Antenatal, delivery and postnatal comparisons of maternal satisfaction with two pilot Changing Childbirth schemes compared with a traditional model of care. *Midwifery.* 2001; **17**: 123–32.

29 Hundley V, Penney G, Fitzmaurice A, *et al.* A comparison of data obtained from service providers and service users to assess the quality of maternity care. *Midwifery.* 2002; **18**: 126–35.

30 Green J, Baston H. Feeling in control during labour: concepts, correlates and consequences. *Birth.* 2003; **30**(4): 235–47.

31 Jomeen J, Martin CR. The impact of choice of maternity care on psychological health outcomes for women during pregnancy and the postnatal period. *J Eval Clin Pract.* 2008; **14**(3): 391–8.

32 Renfrew MJ, Green JM, Spiby H. *Evidence Submitted to the House of Commons Health Committee Maternity Sub-committee 1st Inquiry (2003:03).* Mother and Infant Research Unit: University of Leeds.

33 Beech B. Challenging the illusion of choice. *AIMS.* 2003; **15**(3): 1.

34 Mander R. *Caesarean: just another way of birth.* Abingdon: Routledge; 2007.

35 Edwards NP. *Birthing Autonomy: women's experiences of planning home births.* Abingdon: Routledge; 2005.

36 Beake S, Bick D. Maternity Services Policy: does the rhetoric meet the reality. *Br J Midwifery.* 2007; **14**(10): 609–13.

37 Kitzinger S. *Birth Crisis.* Abingdon: Routledge; 2006.

38 Walker J. Women's experiences of transfer from a midwife led to a consultant led maternity unit in the UK during late pregnancy and labour. *J Midwifery Wom Health.* 2000; **45**(2): 161–8.

39 Gatrell C. *Hard Labour: the sociology of parenthood.* Maidenhead: Open University Press; 2005.

40 Lavender T, Walkinshaw SA, Walton I. A prospective study of women's views of factors contributing to a positive birth experience. *Midwifery.* 1999; **15**: 40–6.

41 Schneider Z. An Australian study of women's experiences of their first pregnancy. *Midwifery.* 2002; **18**: 238–49.

42 Davies Floyd RE. *Birth as an American Rite of Passage.* California: University of California Press; 1992.

43 Maushart S. *The Mask of Motherhood.* Sydney: Vintage; 1997.

44 Slade P, MacPherson SA, Hume A, *et al.* Expectations, experiences and satisfaction with labour. *Br J Clin Psychol.* 1993; **32**: 469–83.

45 Oakley A. *Essays on Women, Medicine and Health.* Edinburgh: Edinburgh University Press; 1993.

46 Milan M. Childbirth as healing; three women's experience of independent midwife care. *Compl Ther Nurs Midwifery.* 2003; **9**: 140–6.

47 Edwards NP. Women planning homebirths: their own views on their relationships with their midwives. In: Kirkham M, editor. *The Midwife-Mother Relationship.* Basingstoke: Palgrave Macmillan; 2000.

48 DiMatteo MR, Khan KL, Berry SH. Narratives of birth and the postpartum: analysis of the focus group responses of new mothers. *Birth*. 1993; **20**: 204–11.

49 Eakins P. *The American Way of Birth*. Philadelphia: Temple University Press; 1996.

50 Cunningham JD. Experiences of Australian mothers who gave birth either at home, at a birth centre, or in hospital labour wards. *Soc Sci Med*. 1993; **36**(4): 475–83.

51 Martin CR, Jomeen J. The impact of clinical management type on maternal locus of control in pregnant women with pre-labour rupture of membranes at term. *Health Psychology Update*. 2004; **13**: 3–13.

52 Brewin C, Bradley C. Perceived control and the experience of childbirth. *Br J Clin Psychol*. 1982; **21**: 263–9.

53 Anderson T. Feeling safe enough to let go: the relationship between a woman and her midwife during the second stage of labour. In: Kirkham M, editor. *The Midwife-Mother Relationship*. Basingstoke: Palgrave Macmillan; 2000.

54 Gould D. Quality care is more than a set of processes. *Br J Midwifery*. 2009; **17**(4): 210.

55 Czarnocka AJ, Slade P. Prevalence and predictors of posttraumatic stress symptoms following childbirth. *Br J Clin Psychol*. 2000; **39**: 35–51.

56 Scott-Palmer J, Skevington SM. Pain during childbirth and menstruation: a study of locus of control. *J Psychosom Res*. 1981; **25**: 151–5.

57 Tinsley BJ, Trupin SR, Owens L, *et al*. The significance of women's pregnancy related locus of control beliefs for adherence to recommended prenatal health regimens and pregnancy outcomes. *J Reprod Infant Psychol*. 1993; **11**: 97–102.

58 Lowe NK. Self-efficacy for labour and childbirth fears in nulliparous pregnant women. *Psychosom Obstet Gynocol*. 2000; **21**(4): 219–24.

59 Wallston KA, Wallston BS, Devellis R. Development of the Multidimensional Health Locus of Control (MHLC) scales. *Health Educ Monog*. 1978; **6**: 160–70.

60 DiMatteo MR, Khan KL. In: Gallant SJ, Puryear KG, Royal Schaler R, editors. *Health Care for Women: psychological, social and behavioural influence*. Washington, DC: American Psychological Association; 1997.

CHAPTER 2

Competing discourses in maternity care

The historical context of childbirth and its link to the subordination of women more generally is well documented and referred to throughout the literature on pregnancy and birth[1,2,3] and it is not necessarily useful to reproduce that in detail again here. It is, however, important to highlight some of the key discourses to which women are exposed as they plan and experience their pregnancies and negotiate their maternity experience. There is acknowledged and often open conflict between obstetricians and midwives, and more recently with women themselves. Kent suggests that this is more a conflict about who knows best and about different views of pregnancy and childbirth. It is an exercise in the ability to exercise power in order to influence and shape services, rather than about fundamental ideologies as such.[4]

BIRTH AS 'NORMAL'

The discourses around birth as a natural and normal biological and physiological process rather than a pathological one have seen a resurgence over the last two decades. The influential birth consumer movement, which began in the 1970s, contested the medicalisation of childbirth and the homogenising of women, highlighting how pregnancy and birth practices stereotyped women as incapable of knowing their own bodies and making their own decisions.[5]

Authors have highlighted a tendency in some criticisms of medical management of labour to hark back to a 'golden age of childbirth' suggesting we should be mindful of conceptualising normal childbirth as inherently safe.[4] Indeed, there is an inherent political element at play that cannot be ignored, where midwives have perceived caesarean sections and medicalisation more broadly as a threat to their role within the reproduction and childbearing arena.

An increased emphasis on normal childbearing as the domain and remit of midwives has been one of the responses to the threat,[6] but what is clear is that a palpable subjectivity of the meaning of normality remains.

Despite the fact that the word 'normal' has been used in relation to labour and birth for centuries, a number of differing definitions and interpretations exist. The difficulty with normal is that it is most often interpreted in the context of the most common or usual outcome.[7] Most frequently it is taken to mean a low-risk physiological labour and a vaginal birth with no or minimal intervention.[7] The World Health Organization (WHO)[8] and the Royal College of Midwives focus on spontaneous onset of labour as a defining element of normality, and highlight other aspects that minimise intervention such as intermittent ausculta-tion, alternative pain relief and spontaneous vertex delivery. The normal delivery definition adopted within government statistics is birth without caesarean, assisted delivery, induction of labour or regional anaesthesia.[7] Walsh identifies that a consensus working definition of normal labour has now been agreed and excludes epidural or spinal anaesthesia, forceps or ventouse, caesarean section and episiotomy but claims that the fact that it does not include other factors such as augmentation and induction of labour, electronic fetal monitoring, an active third stage and opiod use demonstrates compromise.[9] The paradox here is that women with an epidural, for example, may achieve many of the other aspects that are consistent with a normal birth definition, such as spontaneous onset of labour and a vaginal birth, which may lead to the lucid personal assumption that their experience has been 'normal' yet within the definitions above, could not be considered so. Despite the WHO's definition of 'normal birth' clearly excluding such women they also acknowledge that 'the labour and delivery of many high risk pregnant women have a normal course' (p. 8).[8]

Mander offers a hopeful meaning of normal which aims to provide food for thought; she suggests intervention free as a useful term, which by its very nature precludes operative and instrumental birth.[10] However, the crucial factor that such a definition hinges on concerns what constitutes an intervention. Gould's concept analysis of how the term normal labour could be used proposes many aspects that concur with the definitions outlined above, those that differ include 'upright', linked to the woman's posture in physiological labour; 'healthy' and 'natural', which whilst synonymous with normality also remain broadly unde-fined.[11] Mander, however, terms the use of the word healthy as unhelpful because while all births should be maintained within the bounds of good health this is not always through physiological means.[10]

Gould does, however, highlight the potential for 'normal' to become the ideal for which women then strive.[11] Defining normal childbirth may indeed pose a key question about how normality is defined by women in a contemporary context. Is normality defined by outcome or by process? Whilst the lobbying for a return to the conceptualisation of birth as a normal event, and recognition that there is physiological variation between women rather than a homogenised average,[12] has many advantages for women and practitioners, further fundamental questions arise. If homogeneous elements define a normal birth, then the critique directed at the medicalised model of maternity care can equally be applied to a defined model of normality. More importantly what does this mean for women who as Gould[11] suggests strive for the ideal and fail to meet it – have they experienced an 'abnormal birth' and what then are the consequences for that group of women who fail to meet the homogenised standard of normality?

Rigidly defining normal birth and promoting it as the optimal experience risks engendering those women who do not achieve birth within that definition, with a sense of loss. In their book on caesarean birth in Britain, Churchill, Savage and Francombe report the comments of women who had undergone caesarean sections, both planned and emergency.[13] Women's comments include words such as guilty, disappointed, upset, shocked and let down. Women talked about how they would have preferred a normal delivery and the guilt that ensued as a result of not giving birth normally.

However, it is important to note that women also used words such as safer, live-saving and relieved, highlighting how despite initial desires for a 'normal birth' experience and choices that might facilitate these are often secondary to concerns about the ultimate well-being of their baby.[13] Kitzinger has highlighted how women act out of fear of not following professional advice, particularly when the majority of interventions are explained in terms of benefits to the baby.[14] This leads us intuitively to consider the discourses that women are exposed to of birth as risky, which will be addressed in the next section.

Sue Downe has proposed the potential of salutogenesis, as an outcome measure for birth and a way of maximising the potential for optimum birthing.[15] Salutogenesis in opposition to iatrogenesis (which means harm caused directly by supposedly therapeutic interventions) focuses on the generation of well-being, considering health and how to promote it rather than illness and how to cure it, hence it is a process inevitably entangled with and modelled by socio-cultural factors of the individual, the family and their community. Downe and McCourt describe salutogenic well-being as an end product of complex, personal and societal interactions, which has the ability to invert the risk approach to childbirth. They further suggest that rather than a list of conditions and social situations which rule out a physiological birth, the idea of positive forces allows a woman to bring salutogenic aspects of her clinical, emotional, social, spiritual and family history into the birth experience.[16] Such an approach sees neither the privileging of the technological or the physiological, but acknowledges the uniqueness of each woman's circumstances, prioritising and maximising positive well-being as the primary approach. This inevitably leads to a position where normal labour cannot be a catch-all definition or even a category, a flexible definition of normality is necessary, which maximises the possibility of a physiological birth but also optimises the experience of intervention for those women who require it,[16] and potentially diminishes the potential for feelings of failure and distress associated with failure to achieve the 'gold standard' of normality. Evidence has demonstrated that when the concept of salutogenesis is embedded as a philosophy for women prior to birth it had an impact on birthing practices in particular the use of epidural analgesia.[17] However, the concept of salutogenesis, whilst overtly supported by the Royal College of Midwives, is not, as evidence has demonstrated, embedded in obstetric or even midwifery practice,[12] adding to the confusion amongst the profession about what defines normality in terms of birth. It can be assumed that such a lack of consistency can only lead to confusion amongst women themselves regarding the definition of normality.

BIRTH AS A 'RISKY EVENT'

Historically pregnancy and birth was a risky business and rarely viewed with the excitement and anticipation that it is today. In the eighteenth century, maternal mortality and morbidity was high and poor pregnancy outcomes were commonplace. Oakley argues that the idea of pregnancy at this time was a natural one and nature was the judge of its management and outcome,[18] hence beyond the control of women themselves but also beyond the control of experts.[19] During the late 1800s the percentage of women delivering in hospitals was only 1%.[20] However, by the early 1900s modern capitalist states began to take a serious interest in health and welfare. Governments became preoccupied with reduction of mortality and a furtherance of all dimensions of health. Infant mortality was seen as preventable and thus became a focus for policy makers, making children the objects of medical discourse.[21] Initially medical surveillance covered childbirth and child health and then a more sophisticated epidemiology brought medical attention to the prenatal period, coinciding with a new priority, the prevention of maternal death. From the 1920s there was an increased emphasis on hospital birth and over time the direct association between increased hospitalisation and fall in perinatal mortality was constructed. This scientifically constructed discourse ignored all the other socio-economic factors at play[22] and the impact of the wider changes in women's circumstances as significant in improving perinatal outcomes.[23,24] Tew has argued vociferously that the correlations claimed by the medical profession to underpin obstetric practices were clearly spurious,[3] failing to demonstrate causality between medical interventions and falling mortality rates. She observes that the belief that physical science holds adequate insight into the reproductive process provides an erroneous basis for obstetric intervention.[4] Despite such critiques and a general acknowledgement by the 1990s that encouraging all women to give birth in hospital could not be justified on the grounds of safety or as a basis for what had become routine obstetric interventions, increasing and embedded use of technology had created a spiral of rising expectations and the seeds were sown.

Poor outcomes in the developed world are now relatively rare, women seek advice and support from early in the pregnancy and problems can then be detected and addressed. Such an approach has, it has been argued, led to managed pregnancies where risk is significantly lessened; Gross and Pattison suggest, however, that this has not been matched by a reduction in the expectations of risk.[19] The pre-industrial notion of pregnancy and birth being pre-shaped and controlled by nature has been replaced by notions of human agency in pregnancy and individual and social responsibility to manage the potential risks that may occur. Writing on the 'risk society,' Ulrich Beck suggests that physical risks are created by social systems, organisations and institutions which then manage that risky activity.[25] Lupton's philosophy of risk incorporates a secularised approach to life where things don't just happen but can be predicated.[26] The essence of risk is not what is happening but what might happen or be happening. Risk construction must obey the discourse of its revelation and the media and the professions in charge of defining risk become the key players. Hence, science determines risk and the population perceives risk. Risk ultimately then depends on decisions made.[25] Debates about safety in obstetrics have emerged from the epidemiological evidence, however tenuous, regarding maternal mortality and morbidity as well as perinatal deaths.[4] Despite the theoretical and methodological concerns about the evidence which underpins the premise of safety, women continue to perceive medically-defined risks as real, frequently propagated by the mass media, to assess their own pregnancies and make the 'right choices to reduce risk'. Authors have illustrated a collapse of confidence among women, particularly primigravid women about their ability to birth without routine intervention.[27,28] Walsh highlights the alarming intervention rates in low-risk first birth women in the UK.[12]

In an industrialised society, options and choices are greater but so are the demands and expectations on an individual. What seems imperative to pregnant women is to give their unborn child the best chance of being healthy and 'normal' so that they will be able to compete and succeed in modern society. Within maternity care freedom of choice is proclaimed, but the momentum of technology and the clever packaging of the evidence with its focus on monitoring and detecting problems appears compulsive within the concept of responsibility and results in medically-defined right choices.[29]

COMMODIFICATION OF PREGNANCY AND BIRTH

Women are now portrayed as consumers of maternity services and the commodification of birthing, which is seen in the purchase of baby equipment such as the 'right pram' and co-ordinated nursery equipment. This context is largely media driven and assisted by the consumer culture in which we now live, where certain purchases are seen as essential to motherhood. However, this now extends to choice and to making decisions for maternity care, and the commodification of the experience chosen. Kightley suggests that:

> this commodification may extend to the experience of coming into hospital, getting on to a bed, being monitored, being scanned, vaginal examinations, identity bands for mother and for baby, Bounty bags and countless other commodities and rituals. Media portrayals also hold out the promise of emergency procedures, overworked but dedicated teams of staff and machines that go 'beep' if one attends hospital for birth. These images and expectations are also part of our culture and tradition of birthing and women may feel short-changed if they haven't been close to, or even received such intervention (p. 477).[30]

Kightley is proposing that women buy into a certain expected experience of birth in a hospital setting.[30] Conversely considering women who chose a birth-centre delivery may not necessarily be making a choice for type of birth they want per se but rather for the whole experience that birthing in such an environment brings. Indeed, the ambience of birth centres has been cited as central to women's decisions to choose to give birth there.[12] Birth centres often provide a more intimate environment and context for birth, Kirkham suggests that within small-scale maternity care settings relationships are very different.[29] One possible interpretation of a woman's choice for a birth-centre experience could be that women feel they are getting a better level of care or increased value for money. Such choices also potentially link back to the earlier discussion of normal birth as the ideal toward which many women now strive; choice of birth centre may be perceived by women as consuming a philosophy of birth and maximising the potential of reaching the gold standard birth outcome.[31] Whilst the evidence insinuates that assumptions cannot be made about the philosophies or practises of midwives who work in birth centres,[12] women believe they are buying into a certain experience.

Antenatal scanning provides a prime example of a commodified aspect of pregnancy. Ultrasound scanning offered as part of antenatal care is a screening intervention and whilst it has been demonstrated to be anxiety provoking,[32] research supports its value to women in terms of both visual confirmation of the pregnancy and pleasure.[33] Scanning generally has been welcomed by parents as an opportunity to see the fetus and as such is now an integral part of the pregnancy experience. It provides a visibility to the fetus through which it turns into a baby. 3D and 4D scanning is a relatively new option to the maternity care marketplace, offering pregnant couples the opportunity to view a 3D real-time image of their fetus. The imaging benefits of 3D scanning have been documented. However, within the UK, technology is not broadly utilised in a screening context or as part of routine antenatal care but is offered as a consumer experience. The private companies who offer this service promote the experience, in terms of parental-fetal attachment and prenatal bonding, experiences inherently associated with a positive pregnancy experience and successful future parenting. The offering of such services for a fee suggests that there is an experience of pregnancy, in this case a relationship with the baby that can be acquired through a purchased experience.

Symon eloquently raises the ethical component of consumerism and choice within maternity care.[34] It can be argued that, in a payment for care model as available outside the UK, choices can be made as for any other area of economic activity. Does that mean a woman should be able to pay for options such as caesarean section when there is no clinical indication? It may be thought that such as debate is not as yet significantly relevant in the UK. Whilst there is a growing perception that the number of women requesting a caesarean without medical need is increasing, the actual figures are largely unknown because of the complexity of the negotiation and decision-making process.[10] Little is known about the rationale of maternal request for caesarean section.[35] It is entirely possible that requests for an elective caesarean section without clinical indication are influenced by current trends and their profile in the media. Mander highlights the role of the media in reporting on those celebrities who request birth by caesarean, and have their requests granted despite no obvious medical indication, as a significant influence to women, reinforcing societal discourses of birth as inherently risky and promoting a caesarean as the way to avoid the risk.[10] In conjunction with the earlier discussion on the risk discourse surrounding pregnancy this highlights just one of the many complexities of the choice debate. Rhetoric of choice for maternity care could underpin the notion that a woman has positive rights to demand an intervention that is available in the maternity marketplace as well as to refuse an intervention.

SUMMARY

As women are offered the choice in maternity care, they are surrounded by a plethora of culturally established discourses and societal norms. Some of these discourses, such as the birth as risky discourse, are clearly more embedded than others, for instance the more recent commodification of pregnancy and birth discourse. The evidence that has been discussed appears to suggest that these more embedded discourses to date, have seemed to be influential on choice in maternity care. Further, the different discourses to which women are subject are at times in open opposition to each other, and how women make sense of them in such a context with particular reference to choice remains more ambiguous. Whilst the influential nature of some of these discourses has previously been documented, the women's stories that are told here will enlighten further how women are enabled or restricted in choice and decision-making. These women will furnish an appreciation of how they themselves acknowledge, interpret, accept or reject those influential aspects when making choices in maternity care.

REFERENCES

1 Oakley A. *Women Confined: towards a sociology of childbirth.* Oxford: Martin Robinson; 1980.
2 Donnison J. *Midwives and Medical Men: a history of the struggle for the control of childbirth.* London: Historical Publications; 1988.
3 Tew M. *Safer Childbirth? A Critical History of Maternity Care.* London: Chapman & Hall; 1992.
4 Kent J. *Social Perspectives on Pregnancy and Childbirth for Midwives, Nurses and the Caring Professions.* Buckingham: Open University Press; 2000.
5 Kitzinger J. Strategies of the early childbirth movement: a case-study of the National Childbirth Trust. In: Garcia J, Fitzpatrick R, Richards M, editors. *The Politics of Maternity Care: services for childbearing women in twentieth-century Britain.* Oxford: Oxford University Press; 1990.
6 Mander R. *Caesarean: just another way of birth.* Abingdon: Routledge; 2007.
7 Beech BL, Phipps B. Normal birth: women's stories. In: Downe S, editor. *Normal Childbirth: evidence and debate.* Philadelphia: Churchill Livingstone; 2004.
8 World Health Organization. *Care in Normal Birth: a practical guide,* 1996. Available at www.who.int/reproductivehealth/publications/maternal_perinatal_health/MSM_96_24_/en/index.html (accessed 30/03/10).
9 Walsh D. Pain and epidural use in labour. *Evidence Based Midwifery.* 2009; 7(3). Available at www.rcm.org.uk/ebm/ebm-2009/september-2009/pain-and-epidural-use-in-normal-childbirth (accessed 12/12/09).
10 Mander R. *Caesarean: just another way of birth.* Abingdon: Routledge; 2007.
11 Gould D. Normal labour: a concept analysis. *J Adv Nurs.* 2000; 31(2): 418–27.
12 Walsh D. *Evidence-based Care for Normal Labour and Birth: a guide for midwives.* Abingdon: Routledge; 2007.

13 Churchill H, Savage W, Francome C. *Caesarean Birth in Britain: a book for health professionals and parents.* Enfield: Middlesex University Press; 2006.

14 Kitzinger S. *Birth Crisis.* Abingdon: Routledge; 2006.

15 Downe S. Defining normal birth. *MIDRS Midwifery Digest.* 2001; **11**(suppl 2): S31–S33.

16 Downe S, McCourt C. From being to becoming: reconstructing childbirth knowledges. In: Downe S, editor. *Normal Childbirth: evidence and debate.* Philadelphia: Churchill Livingstone; 2004.

17 Foster J. Innovative practice in birth education. In: Nolan M, Foster J, editors. *Birth and Parenting Skills: new directions in antenatal education.* London: Elsevier; 2005.

18 Oakley A. *The Captured Womb: a history of the medical care of pregnant women.* 2nd ed. Oxford: Basil Blackwell; 1986.

19 Gross H, Pattison H. *Sanctioning Pregnancy.* Hove: Routledge; 2007.

20 Foster P. *Women and the Healthcare Industry: an unhealthy relationship.* Buckingham: Open University Press; 1995.

21 Oakley A. Doctors, maternity patients and social scientists. *Birth.* 1985; **12**:161–6.

22 Beech B. *Penalities of Obstetric Technology.* Buckinghamshire: AIMS; 1992.

23 Doyal L. *What Makes Women Sick: gender and the political economy of health.* Basingstoke: Open University Press; 1995.

24 Hunt S, Symonds A. *The Social Meaning of Midwifery.* Basingstoke: Macmillan Press; 1995.

25 Beck U. *Risk Society: towards a new modernity.* London: Sage; 1992.

26 Lupton D. *The Imperative of Health.* London: Sage; 1995.

27 Downe S, McCormick C, Beech B. Labour interventions associated with normal birth. *Br J Midwifery.* 2001; **9**(10): 602–6.

28 Mead M. Midwives perspectives in 11 UK maternity units. In: Downe S, editor. *Normal Childbirth: Evidence and Debate.* Philadelphia: Churchill Livingstone; 2004.

29 Kirkham M. *Informed Choice in Maternity Care.* Basingstoke: Palgrave Macmillan; 2004.

30 Kightley R. Delivering choice: where to birth? *Br J Midwifery.* 2007; **15**(8): 475–8.

31 Coyle K, Hauck Y, Percival P. Normality and collaboration: mothers perceptions of birth centre versus hospital care. *Midwifery.* 2001; **17**(3): 182–93.

32 Green J. *Calming or Harming? A critical review of the psychological effects of fetal diagnosis of pregnant women.* London: Galton Institute; 1990.

33 Larsen T, Nguyen TH, Munk M. Ultrasound screening in the 2nd trimester. The pregnant woman's background, knowledge, expectations and acceptances. *Ultrasound Obstet Gynecol.* 2000; **15**: 383–6.

34 Symon A. *Risk and Choice in Maternity Care: an international perspective.* Philadelphia: Churchill Livingstone; 2006.

35 Lavender T, Kingdon C. Caesarean delivery at maternal request: why we should promote normal birth. *Br J Midwifery.* 2005; **14**(5): 302–3.

CHAPTER 3

Discourses of motherhood

A MOTHERHOOD OR MOTHERING IDENTITY

Only 9% of women never seek or want a pregnancy,[1] suggesting that the majority of women do wish to produce a child and become mothers. Identified drivers for this include achieving some sense of importance and recognised adult status, being truly needed by another human being, which affords an opportunity for exercising power and influence, providing a bridge to the future, diminishing the fear of one's own death and providing an opportunity for the expansion of oneself.[1] Debates have long raged over the biological or socially constructed nature of the mother–child bond. The issues of pregnancy, birth and child rearing became a key focus for feminist writers in the 1970s and 1980s when until that time the image of the homemaking wife and mother had been the dominant cultural depiction and motherhood was constructed as a role firmly within the family context. Adrienne Rich in *Of Woman Born* referred to this construction of motherhood as the patriarchal institution of motherhood that is male-defined, controlled and is deeply oppressive to women, as opposed to mothering, which refers to women's experiences of mothering that are female-defined, centred and potentially empowering.[2] Rich's work identifies both the oppressive and empowering dimensions of maternity and motherhood as well as the complex relationship between the two.[3] Since Rich's early distinctions, many other feminist writers have dedicated themselves to critiquing and demystifying motherhood, ascertaining two competing views. The negative discourse that focuses on motherhood as a social mandate and a compromise of a woman's independence, where the carrying and birthing of children inevitably brings with it the responsibility for all aspects for their upbringing, and the positive discourse which argues that motherhood minus patriarchy has the potential to bond women to their children and to each other, and release a liberating knowledge of the self.[3]

Despite such critiques women remain defined by the notion that normal women become or at least desire to become mothers.[4] Motherhood is considered to be a normative stage of a woman's development, a crucial part of their identity and for some women provides an occupational and structural identity.[5] Early feminist writers have been critiqued for ignoring the primal pull that exists with regard to motherhood,[6] and for many women motherhood continues to be described as a natural progression and ultimately fulfilling.[7]

The transition to motherhood is traditionally conceptualised as the period after giving birth and this is reinforced by literature that considers the impact of motherhood on women's roles, identities and social relations, including those with partners, the wider family and friends, and through employment.[8,9] Theories such as Mercer's maternal role attainment theory,[10] describe pregnancy as an anticipatory stage. Gatrell refers to several sociological writers including Oakley, Cusk and Davidson who all describe birth as the point of transition reinforcing the notion that commencement of the mothering role does not formally begin until after birth.[6]

PREGNANCY AND A MOTHERING IDENTITY

Pregnancy has been represented as a potential crisis state, involving shifts in identity and the move from non-motherhood to motherhood.[11] Acknowledged as a time where a woman prepares for motherhood, by seeking information, visualising herself in the maternal role, demonstrating an attachment to the fetus and the beginning of an emotional bond. It is also a period where women can face a confrontation with unresolved issues such as sexual abuse, previous traumatic birth[12] and poor parenting, all interpretations that continue to suggest pregnancy as the transition stage prior to motherhood. Transition is also a major psychological discourse, recognising pregnancy as a time of emotional change as well as physical. Unfortunately, the basis of such discourse in a bio-medical frame generally highlights the possible deleterious and negative impact of transition on a woman's psychological status.[13]

Realignment of identity occurs within a personal, social and political context and the public visibility of pregnancy permits it to become the focus of public discourse. Discourses, such as the bio-medical model of pregnancy, the psychological aspects of pregnancy and contemporary discourses of choice permit others to comment on the pregnancy and the woman's actions and responses to it. Women themselves reconceptualise themselves as part of a distinct and specific club of like women.[11] As members of this club they are expected to behave in certain ways and within certain boundaries, set by wider discourses, some of which have already been discussed. The metaphor of the pregnant women as a vessel for the fetus at the mercy of elemental forces that may endanger the vessels contents has been presented by feminist writers.[13] Such discourses as well as the biomedical discourse of risk already discussed, expect women to make safe and responsible but informed choices about pregnancy and childbirth that ultimately protect the well-being of the fetus. The public visibility of pregnancy paradoxically requires both passivity and agency, and it is within this arena that women are faced with a redefinition of their self and their identity. This context is further complicated by the fact that the reality of pregnancy can now be confirmed at a much earlier stage. Home testing pregnancy kits are available to detect a pregnancy before a period has even been missed, pregnancy is therefore confirmed long before the signs and symptoms appear. A potential consequence of this is that the woman's engagement with and responsibility for the pregnancy begins much earlier as does the potential relationship with her baby. Gross and Pattison refer to this 'as being a little bit pregnant'[11] and relate it to Barbara Katz Rothman's influential writing on the 'tentative pregnancy'.[14] The pregnancy becomes a reality at a gestation where it also carries a greater risk of loss. Loss of the pregnancy can then be attributed to personal behaviours, for example consuming alcohol or eating the wrong foods, and be perceived as a personally avoidable mistake. Early loss often happens before contact with healthcare professionals or the maternity system, making responsibility for outcome entirely the woman's with no one else to devolve accountability to.

> The pregnancy test is just one of the first of many tests which will lead to decisions about whether the pregnancy should continue or not (p. 17).[11]

Pregnant women renegotiate their identities within discourses that privilege mothering and deny women identities and selfhood outside motherhood.[7,15] Even those women who do not become mothers are often defined in relation to them as potential mothers through descriptors such as 'childless' and 'infertile' and images of pregnancy and childbirth construct the pregnant woman as made whole.[4] Motherhood is frequently idealised and women's accounts describe becoming a mother as ultimately fulfilling.[16] Western concepts of motherhood emphasise attachment, nurturing and intense fulfilling emotions, all of which are associated with the natural attributes of women.[17,18] It is by these standards that mothering practices are evaluated. Mothering consists of historically and culturally variable practices of nurturing and caring for dependent children. The practice of mothering is constructed in specific circumstances and is consistent with prevailing cultural beliefs. 'The ideology of intensive mothering' described by Hays, declared mothering as exclusive, wholly child centred, emotionally involving and time consuming.[19] The mother portrayed here is devoted to the care of others and self-sacrificing, intensive mothering acts as the dominant cultural script and reinforces a gendered female identity.[17,18] Mothers who do not conform to the normative standard against which all mothering practices are judged, are affected in that their practices are evaluated by it and even those who contest it are immersed in it.[20] Prescriptions about how 'good mothers' behave provide the framework for evaluating the practices and behaviours of others.

The social policy discourse celebrates women's 'natural' abilities and understands good mothering as the key to a child's successful development, placing the responsibility and the onus on the mother. This is consistent with the expectations placed on pregnant women. Both pregnant women and mothers consult expertise and 'engage in reflexive encounters with expert systems'[17] to make responsible decisions about the development of their children (and fetuses). Glenn suggests that women are powerful figures in children's lives giving them a valued position and role, although this is often experienced as blame when things do not turn out right.[7] This corresponds to the blame attributed to women who do not make the right decisions in pregnancy or behave in the right way, for example women who refuse screening can be construed as irresponsible.[21] Motherhood is construed as problematic for those women who do not bring children up in the right circumstances,[15] as is a pregnancy defined by a medical model that emphasises women's instrumental role in a successful, problem free pregnancy. The 'identification of a fetus as a potentially healthy baby could be interpreted as a means by which women are encouraged to adopt responsible behaviours' (p. 298).[11]

Authors have discussed the importance of the 'maternal instinct' as one that naturalises maternity and continues to influence contemporary attitudes towards motherhood and mothering, despite the arguments which have raged against such a conceptualisation. Kitzenger describes how birth fundamentally changes a woman's identity and that she becomes a different kind of person, that is to say a mother.[4] Other authors such as Oakley have, however, suggested the idea that pregnancy automatically triggers a maternal response.[22]

THE INSTITUTION OF MOTHERHOOD

Only four to five decades ago the image of a mother was one who stayed at home and was identified by her role as a housewife and mother, a role that was very definitely within the family setting.[6] As recently as the 1980s Ann Oakley commented on the challenge inherent in becoming a mother where women were only able to have a professional job or a baby but not both.[23] The notion of the perfect and selfless mother continued to be a pervasive socially constructed institution of motherhood. It can be argued that those societal constructions have moved on, helped by the equality and diversity agenda and mandate, with the rising number of female workers the most obvious indication of the changing context for women. Over the last four decades 'the image of the nondomestic woman has emerged to challenge the predominance of the homemaker-mother' (p. 8),[24] which has been claimed by some writers to challenge the dominance of the traditional household. However, old tensions remain and new tensions emerge. The traditional roles of wife and mother continue to be emphasised by some writers and the domestic woman still undoubtedly exists.[24] In addition, there is now a current and acknowledged tension between those mothers who choose to stay at home and 'career mothers', with both working women and career mothers reporting undertones of disapproval at their choices.[24,25] The media periodically presents research findings that consider the impact of working, or of the effect of leaving children in childcare, on children's short- and long-term outcomes in behavioural and intellectual terms, which is more often than not presented as a damaging one. Women who choose to continue to work, particularly those who pursue a career, and often told they cannot 'have it all', although some authors report that there is no 'having it all' dream.[26] Conversely, mothers who choose not to work report feeling social and financial pressure to return to work. In essence what this achieves is little more than to reinforce the notion that it is an either/or choice between a career and motherhood.

These discussions and debates are particularly influential to women in the postnatal period following the birth of their babys. They are inherently linked to the public assumption, perhaps in part a legacy from pregnancy, that it is acceptable to judge women's mothering practices and abilities. Compared to the support that they have previously received in pregnancy the postnatal period is a time when support is withdrawn relatively quickly and women are left in comparative isolation, a situation that can render women segregated, lonely and often feeling inadequate.

The last two decades has seen a new phenomenon emerge in which expert advice is directed at women through a plethora of parenting texts and magazines as well as virtual information via the internet.[6] These many texts contain directives that are addressed to women, and contain prescriptive messages about a certain lifestyle and about how good mothers behave.[26] These parenting texts construct a notion of 'instant love', which is automatic and natural and also an essential ingredient of motherhood,[27] hence mothers who cannot ascribe those feelings to their own experience are by default abnormal and failing in some way. It has been suggested that these parenting guides are most likely to affect well-educated, middle-class, older first-time mums. Gatrell suggests that these are the women who are most likely to professionalise the institution of motherhood.[6] However, it seems feasible to suggest that these expert theories of child rearing provide a potentially oppressive foundation to all women entering motherhood.[28]

Most expert manuals assume the presence of a father and instruct the mother on what his role should be, indeed mothers are required to mediate the relationship between the father and the baby and balance the individual needs of family members against the family as a unit.[6] The powerful and significant message within this implies that a mother's desire to have a life of her own outside the family endangers the family unit.

DOMESTIC LABOUR

Ann Oakley observed that motherhood entails a great deal of domestic work.[23] Gatrell identifies substantial evidence supporting the notion that though much may have changed in terms of the likelihood of women having a career in conjunction with child rearing; that they continue to also carry the responsibility of domestic labour has not changed, irrespective of the nature or demands of the work that they do.[6] There is some evidence of changes in the division of household labour and confirmation does exist to suggest that husbands/partners now do more housework.[29] The radical feminist writer Christine Delphy, however, contends that beyond household labour women also carry the onus of supporting their husbands/partners careers. She suggests that this is in part due to societal expectations of employers that female partners will assist male employees in their working lives, 'whilst the wage-labourer sells his labour power, the married woman gives hers away', and she further highlights that this expectation is unlikely to be reciprocated.[30] Maushart refers to this phenomenon, which also includes a responsibility for domestic labour, as 'wifework' and argues that those who recoil from such responsibility are termed as selfish. She further emphasises that while intellectually society rejects the idea of 'wifework', emotionally and behaviourally it remains pervasive and the old male-oriented paradigm remains entrenched.[31] The further implications of this, according to Maushart are that fathers (even the most loving) take little overall responsibility for childcare, his responsibilities relative to his wife will remain focused on his role as financial provider and hence, for the most part, abstract. These authors assert that women remain charged with overall responsibility for domestic labour, for childcare and routine childcare tasks even in the face of the most helpful husband. More recent work suggests that little has changed with regard to the domestic division of labour, an expectation that may be particularly intimidating for mothers as they aspire to perfection.[6] Ozer recently explored the impact of childcare responsibility on the psychological health of professional working mothers and found that that greater childcare responsibility is associated with lower well-being and greater psychological distress. However, both well-being and distress are consistently mediated by a woman's belief in her capability to enlist the help of her spouse for childcare.[32] It is noteworthy that this theory does not lessen a woman's responsibility, seemingly continuing to invest women with the ultimate accountability for childcare. Stevens and colleagues found, however, that marital satisfaction for women was linked to satisfaction with division of labour, which does not imply that an equal split of all domestic labour is essential but more that a mutually agreed division of domestic labour, perceived as fair is important.[33]

It seems viable to consider if Maushart's arguments might extend to the social arena and leisure time, with men often able to link social activity to the furtherance of career prospects. A study utilising Canadian data has indeed demonstrated that mothers had less leisure time than fathers, particularly when children are small, seemingly symptomatic of the primary responsibility for domestic labour that women maintain even in dual-earning couples,[34] although it has also been suggested that active leisure for women is constrained by ideological influences, which would include a commitment to their children.[35] Whilst it has been suggested that women in paid work might feel more entitled to leisure time,[6] other authors have claimed that leisure time declines with increased wages.[36] This association may be explained by the ideological constraints that women report.[35] Hence, analogous to higher work demands and potentially increased time spent at work is guilt,[26] which engenders women with an amplified obligation, in terms of time dedicated to their children and the family rather than to themselves. Notable within these arguments is that many women put themselves at the centre of their family structure,[28] and as such often make employment and life choices that enable them to retain that position and conform to the institution of motherhood.[24,29] This is not the case for all women though and the career women in Caroline Gatrell's study rejected the notion of being identified with the institution of motherhood, although they continued to feel guilty about not being stay-at-home mothers. The notion of guilt that women feel is generally a gender specific phenomenon and studies have identified that working fathers report less family–work conflict and individual stress than working mothers.[37]

Beyond the practical elements essential to family structure is the role that women play in maintaining emotional balance within the home. This includes both the intimate relationship between the mother and the father, and the relationship between the father and the child. It involves resolving and controlling the emotions of other family members and smoothing tensions and strains. This is not merely an abstract concept but a demanding and time-consuming task, which simultaneously is emotionally exacting and requires emotional control on behalf of the mother. The arrival of a baby inevitably changes the relationship among couples, and quality time and shared social activity consequently reduce. Women report investing much of their emotional energy into their children, particularly if they are working mothers, and as a result partner's needs became less of a priority. Interestingly, despite this women still felt a responsibility for the emotional stability of their relationships, leading to a mixture of guilt and resentfulness for what seems an almost impossible task.[6]

SUMMARY

It seems feasible to suggest that the concordance of the characteristics which women display in pregnancy and following birth could potentially blur the pregnant woman and mother dichotomy and question pregnancy as the transition to motherhood phase. Such a conceptualisation would suggest that it is not necessarily birth that is the essential signal which stimulates the maternal caring reaction but, rather, the confirmation of pregnancy. The notion that in contemporary terms pregnancy may be considered the beginning of motherhood will be illuminated by the women who tell their stories within this book. The theoretical significance of this is in its relationship to how women experience maternity encounters, relationships, events, emotions, choice and decision-making.

It appears lucid from the literature on motherhood that women are influenced by the attitudes of others towards their behaviour. This is exceptionally relevant for the women in this book as they negotiate changes in their identities not only following the birth of their babies but across the course of their pregnancies. The construct of the institution of motherhood is a powerful and significant influence to women in terms of how they judge their own abilities, but also in how it creates a climate of opinion against which others perceive women/mothers behaviours and actions. This is of particular relevance if public attitudes suggest a particular action or behaviour is especially beneficial or conversely especially harmful.

The expectations that society places on women through gendered discourses of domestic labour are significant in women's lives and in women's roles within the home, irrespective of their working status. That drivers to 'be perfect' can provoke guilt and that gendered inequities can foster resentment are acutely relevant to the postnatal accounts presented in Part 2 of this book.

REFERENCES

1 Morse CA. Reproduction: a critical analysis. In: Ussher JM, editor. *Women's Health: Contemporary International Health Perspectives.* Leicester: The British Psychological Society; 2000.

2 Rich A. *Of Woman Born: motherhood as an experience and institution.* New York: Norton; 1986.

3 O'Reilly A. *From Motherhood to Mothering.* Albany: State University of New York Press; 2004.

4 Kent J. *Social Perspectives on Pregnancy and Childbirth for Midwives, Nurses and the Caring Professions.* Buckingham: Open University Press; 2000.

5 Phoenix A, Wollett A, Lloyd E. *Motherhood: meanings, practices and ideologies.* London: Sage; 1991.

6 Gatrell C. *Hard Labour: the sociology of parenthood.* Maidenhead: Open University Press; 2005.

7 Glenn EN. Social constructions of mothering: a thematic overview. In: Glenn EN, Chang G, Forcey LR, editors. *Mothering: ideology, experience and agency.* New York: Routledge; 1994.

8 Hakim C. Competing family models, competing social policies. *Family Matters.* 2003; **64**: 52–61.

9 McMahon M. *Engendering Motherhood: identity and self-transformation in women's lives.* New York: The Guilford Press; 1995.

10 Meighan M, Wood A. The impact of hyperemesis gravidarum on maternal role assumption. *J Obstet Gynecol Neonatal Nurs.* 2005; **34**(2): 172–9.

11 Gross, H. Pregnancy: a healthy state. In: Ussher JM, editor. *Women's Health: contemporary international health perspectives.* Leicester: The British Psychological Society; 2000.

12 Kitzinger S. *Birth Crisis.* Abingdon: Routledge; 2006.

13 Gross H, Pattison H. *Sanctioning Pregnancy.* Hove: Routledge; 2007.

14 Katz-Rothman B. *The Tentative Pregnancy: how amniocentesis changes the experience of motherhood.* New York: Viking; 1993.

15 Woollett A, Marshall H. Motherhood and mothering. In: Ussher JM, editor. *Women's Health: contemporary international health perspectives.* Leicester: The British Psychological Society; 2000.

16 Weaver JJ, Ussher JM. How motherhood changes life: a discourse analytical study with mothers of young children. *J Reprod Infant Psychol.* 1997; **15**: 51–68.

17 Vincent C, Ball SJ, Pietikainen S. Metropolitan mothers: mothers, mothering and paid work. *Wom Stud Int Forum.* 2004; **27**: 571–87.

18 Arendell T. Conceiving and investigating motherhood. *J Marriage Fam.* 2000; **62**: 1192–207.

19 Hays S. *The Cultural Contradictions of Motherhood.* New Haven: Yale University Press; 1996.

20 Bell S. Intensive performances of mothering: a sociological perspective. *Qual Res J.* 2004; 4(1): 45–75.

21 Ennis M. Screening: a critique. In: Ussher JM, editor. *Women's Health: Contemporary International Health Perspectives.* Leicester: The British Psychological Society; 2000.

22 Oakley A. *Becoming a Mother.* Oxford: Martin Robertson; 1979.

23 Oakley A. *From Here to Maternity: becoming a mother.* Harmondsworth: Penguin; 1981.

24 Gerson K. *Hard Choices: how women decide about work, career and motherhood.* Los Angeles: University of California Press; 1985.

25 Buxton J. *Ending the Mother War, Starting the Workplace Revolution.* London: McMillan; 1998.

26 Flett K. What having it all means for mums. *The Observer,* 8 November 2009. Available at: www.guardian.co.uk/theobserver/2009/nov/08/kathryn-flett-having-it-all-mothers (accessed 27 February 2010).

27 Marshall H. The social construction of motherhood: an analysis of childcare and parenting manuals. In: Phoenix A, Wollett A, Lloyd E, editors. *Motherhood, Meanings, Practices and Ideologies.* London: Sage; 1991.

28 Ribbens J. *Mothers and Their Children: A Feminist Sociology of Child-rearing.* London: Sage; 1994.

29 Brines J. Economic dependency, gender and the division of labor at home. *Am J Sociol.* 1994; **100**(3): 652–88.

30 Abbott P, Sapsford R. *Women and Social Class.* New York: Tavistock; 1987.

31 Maushart S. *Wifework: what marriage really means for women.* London: Bloomsbury; 2002.

32 Ozer EM. The impact of childcare responsibility and self-efficacy on the psychological health of professional working mothers. *Psychol Women Q.* 2006; **19**(3): 315–35.

33 Stevens D, Kiger G, Riley PJ. Working hard and hardly working: domestic labour and marital satisfaction amongst dual-earner couples. *J Marriage Fam.* 2001; **63**: 514–26.

34 Silver C. Being there: the time dual-earner couples spend with their children. *Canadian Social Trends.* Summer. 2000; p. 9.

35 Brown PR, Brown WJ, Miller YD, Hansen V. Perceived constraints and social support for active leisure among mothers with young children. *Leisure Sci.* 2001; **23**(3): 131–44.

36 Kimmel J, Connelly R. Mothers' time choices: caregiving, leisure, home production, and paid work. *J Hum Resour.* 2007; **62**(3): 643–81.

37 Hill EJ. Work-family facilitation and conflict, working fathers and mothers, work-family stressors and support. *J Fam Issues.* 2005; **26**(6): 793–819.

Summary of Part 1

The chapters above have set the current policy context in relation to choice in maternity care. There has been an explicit attempt to highlight the relationship between choice and control, which may be a vital mechanism for women in terms of how they experience their pregnancy and birth. It is evident that questions still need to be asked about the reality of choice for women.

The notion that pregnancy and childbirth is surrounded by social and cultural constructions, and the belief that women's experiences are situated within and influenced by that context has been explicitly expressed from the outset and is inherent throughout this book. Further societal discourses that traditionally sit outside of pregnancy, such as a mothering identity have been overtly identified as having relevance not only to women's experiences after birth but also to the pregnancy context and in particular how women might approach choice in maternity care.

There is a dominant contemporary rhetoric of woman-centred childbirth, and a strong motivation to encourage women to make choices and decisions about their care. There is a lack of substantive and consistent evidence regarding the multiplicity of factors considered by women in making choices for the management of childbirth. Whilst policy changes imply a move away from the medical discourse of childbirth, robust evidence as to such a change is lacking. It is suggested that the settings and context within which women make choices remain dominated by concerns about risk, risk factors and risk avoidance.

Section two will utilise much of the literature presented in section one to explore and interpret women's pregnancy, childbirth and early motherhood experiences. There will be an overt focus on choice throughout, but this will not be exclusive of the other aspects of their experience, which clearly held importance for women. The interpretations presented will reinforce and extend existing literature, whilst adding a new theoretical dimension to how women encounter their maternity experience.

PART 2

The women's stories

The purpose of Part 2 of this book is to understand the experience of the research participants in the context of the background set out in Part 1. The stories that women tell about their pregnancy and birth experiences within the context of choice will be explored. In order to understand how the interpretations presented in this section have been reached, it seems firstly important to explain how the data produced as a result of the interviews with women was analysed. Some of the following chapter will inevitably present findings that will be revisited in the subsequent chapters. This feels necessary in order to promote a transparent understanding of the analytical journey and of how the final interpretations were reached.

CHAPTER 4

Making sense of the stories told

NARRATIVE AND A SENSE OF SELF

Narrative has been claimed to provide a structure to our sense of selfhood.[1] The stories we tell about our lives to both ourselves and others create a narrative identity by which we recognise ourselves.[1] It is possible to hold a number of different narrative identities, each of which is connected to different social relationships, an aspect which is particularly relevant in the interpretation of the childbirth stories women told. Narrative identity and its connected social relationships, in turn provide a sense of localised coherence and stability.[1] At times of instability, we can make connections to other aspects of our narrative identities. Women in pregnancy and new motherhood are in a process of creating new social relationships defined by both their pregnancy and their baby but also in renegotiating relationships with their partners, family, friends and others. Narrative affords us access to those experiences as described by the women themselves and to how women define themselves at this time in the context of their lives.

The construction of a personal narrative selects the different aspects of our lives and connects them with others, creating a certain order to our lives. This is a process of identity formation that occurs in a changing social and personal context, and the values attached to different experiences in that context influence the character of the events recalled.[1] Though women will tell their stories, the actual structure of the story and the pattern of their lives will be shaped by a multiplicity of social, cultural and psychological forces both conscious and unconscious.[2] Women are active agents who are part of and engage with a social world, and as such their narrative accounts are shaped by social and cultural contexts, as well as the collective narratives that define and distinguish them as pregnant women and mothers from other collective narratives.[1] Collective narratives overlap with personal narratives such that women can define themselves as part of a group as well as individuals. In essence women are enmeshed in a world of narrative; exploration of that narrative allows us access to women's maternity worlds, how they make sense of that world and how they renegotiate their position and identity within it. The following narratives presented highlight the narrative identities that are created by women within their maternity stories. Those identities are shaped by the discourses and influences within women's social and cultural orbits that serve to help create those identities.

Previous studies of motherhood have identified competing discourses of maternity, one the dominant traditional image, the second more subversive and less socially acceptable but a clear product of the women's actual experiences.[3] Coates does not suggest that women are unthinking victims of maternity and motherhood discourses but that their linguistic representations and constructions of their maternity identities will be based on the selection of some discourses and the rejection of others.[3] There is clearly a physical reality and an embodied experience of being pregnant for women but it seems apparent that there is additionally a social and cultural establishment of pregnancy to which women subscribe albeit to differing degrees. The interpretation of women's stories within this book demonstrates how pregnancy and birth shape an individual woman's sense of identity and the reasons why she represents herself by certain narrative constructions either consciously or subconsciously.

INTERPRETING WOMEN'S MATERNITY NARRATIVES

Early interpretation of the stories that women told began with the striking observation of the different ways in which the women in the interviews seemed to be referring to their fetus, i.e. as: 'my baby', 'the baby', 'baby'. An observation went on to provide the key signpost for the analysis of the data.

The fetus never seemed to be referred to as 'our baby' despite the fact that women spoke about trying to get pregnant, and recognised pregnancy as a joint decision and product. The fathers surprisingly in the early pregnancy interviews seemed strangely absent from the women's narratives, yet clearly their role in the pregnancy cannot be denied.

This initial observation actually contradicted the philosophy underpinning much narrative analysis, for rather than what was in the text, in the form of stories being important, what was *not* in the text seemed to offer something equally, if perhaps not more, important. As researchers whilst we sharpen our perception to avoid ascribing meaning to or overwriting our data, at the same time we risk overlooking or ignoring the meaning of what is absent.[4] Paul Ricoeur's hermeneutic theory of interpretation, described in Crotty,[5] offered some useful thoughts regarding interpretation. The *hermeneutics of meaning-recollection* aimed at faithful disclosure of people's life worlds and the *hermeneutics of suspicion*, which aims to discover, behind the thing being analysed, a further reality which allows a much deeper interpretation to be made and which can challenge the surface account.[1] Hermeneutics is defined as a method for deciphering indirect meaning, a reflective practice of unmasking hidden meanings beneath apparent ones. Interpreters may end up with an explicit awareness of meanings that the authors themselves would have been unable to articulate.[5] This approach seemed to offer a method for understanding why women articulate their pregnancy and birth experience in the way that they do and in addition for discovering the meanings they are unable to articulate because they have no language to do so. Ricoeur's analytical framework was not the framework finally applied to the study data. However, the debt to Ricoeur is twofold: the notion that authors' meanings and intentions often remain implicit and go unrecognised by the authors themselves, and the notion that the correct inquiry can allow access to those meanings and intentions that are hidden in the text but unarticulated.

It was then the work of structuralist scholars[6] that further offered ways of thinking about how to analyse voices within the text that are not articulated, alongside those actually being articulated. The final and unique framework for analysis incorporated and combined thematic narrative analysis, the work of A-J Greimas[7,8] on structural analysis, and the work of Rogers, Casey and Ekert[4] on interpretive poetics. The framework developed enabled a focus on narrative identities and enabled illumination of the influential factors that create those identities within women's maternity stories. The following sections aim to capture and present the elements that became key to that analytical framework.

STRUCTURAL ANALYSIS

Structuralist analysis was first described by Propp in 1928.[6] He aimed to classify fairy tales according to their component parts and the relationship of these components to each other. His analysis noted that the same character can perform different actions and different characters may perform the same action. His analysis presented a single structure of seven possible characters and 31 possible actions.[4] The attraction in a structuralist approach was the suggestion that a framework could be developed to identify characters in a narrative and the role/ roles that they could occupy. Later structuralists such as Levi-Strauss praised but critiqued Propp's principles,[9] suggesting that his approach ignored the thematic content inherent in narratives. What structuralism aimed to achieve was to find common cultural elements that would identify universal structures ultimately embedded deep in the human mind. Human beings are the effect of these structures that escape their awareness.[9] In 1966, A-J Greimas (translated 1983) published *Structural Semantics*, which utilised the principals of both Propp and Levi Stauss and provided a key element of the analytical framework.[7]

Greimas utilised Propp's work to develop a model for understanding the organising principles of all narrative discourses and the work of Levi-Strauss highlighting how narrative characters can play multiple roles.[6] Not dissimilar from Ricoeur, Greimas distinguished between a discursive level and a narrative level, between the ways a narrative is told and the narrative itself.

Greimas suggests that a grammatical subject might or might not reveal itself as a person. His model for analysis allowed not only human beings but also animals, objects or concepts to accomplish or undergo an act within the narrative. Building on the initial observations of how the women referred to the fetus, Greimas's concept offered the potential to capture the role of the fetus within the woman's narratives; does the fetus acquire a character of its own or create a character for the woman within her narratives? The fetus has generally been assigned a passive role within women's pregnancy experience but it was potentially feasible to think that the fetus is more than just the object of somebody else's actions, e.g. the pregnant woman, but that it is actually invested of its own agency within the woman's narratives. An additional question was whether the fetus's role changes as the pregnancy progresses, as it certainly does following birth? Adopting this concept offered a way to discover who or what was important and influential to women throughout their maternity narratives. This approach opened up the possibility that key influences could be defined in the women's narratives and may play roles that hold differing importance at different times. It offered the potential to reveal not only the main characters of the woman's narratives but also provided a way of giving a more important place to those non-human influences in the story. It raised the possibility of maternity discourses as significant influences within the women's stories, or at least of characters within the stories told shaped and produced out of cultural and societal discourse. The questions to ask of the women's narratives therefore became, who are the important characters of the piece and how are those characters revealed? Of particular resonance was the notion that one actor can perform more than one role offering the potential for the woman as an intersection of a matrix of influences, which then may reveal more than one identity. This is coherent with both the theory of competing discourses of maternity, but also with my interest in narrative identities and the creation of a dominant narrative identity that the woman chooses to reveal, alongside those that she either consciously or subconsciously represses. Women's experiences and the subsequent emotions and responses aroused clearly seemed to need to express something more than the spoken narrative would allow. An example of this early analysis within the themes illustrates how something more than was actually being articulated seemed to be emerging. The bracketed annotation denotes the tentative early analysis.

'[Y]es yes going back to last question actually it is something you do worry about things going wrong definitely its . . . and now I can feel it [still not referred to as a baby] moving around all the time. [The baby has a physical presence – this reality causes fear about the fact that things may go wrong, and the role of mother/protector has already begun in the conscious noticing of the reduction in movements] I notice that if it hasn't done for a while I'm consciously waiting for it to do so but I know its probably part and parcel of what's natural isn't it? [I: mm yes its become real to you now hasn't it, its like there's no going back now] Absolutely yeah that's definitely happened in the last month'.

'[M]m yeah . . . I suppose that's something else I thought I'd feel more attached than I do I guess [guilt that feelings are not as strong as they should be – who sets the standard?] . . . but I am in that I'm making sure I do everything right I try and sort of do the right things and I'm talking to it and I'm trying to imagine he or she as a person [wants to see her baby as an existing being but finding it difficult because this is someone she doesn't yet know but feels that she should] and erm this kind of thing [good mothering begins early – attending not just to physical well-being of the baby but also to emotional well-being by talking to it] [I: mm mm] but I think C is more, he's more emotionally bonding already [this suggests that M feels she is not emotionally bonding] [I: mm] than I am he'll sit and talk but you see I thought when I first started to feel it move I thought I'd be absolutely overwhelmed with this that's my baby [this is the first time that she actually refers to the fetus as a baby] you know and it hasn't been quite that intense . . . [physical movement makes the baby a reality but the intangibility of the baby seems to make it difficult for M to make the emotional bonds that she feels she should] but I think that will maybe come more gradually for me [I: yeah, yeah and I don't think that's abnormal because it's the first time you're experiencing everything] [she doesn't really know how to feel and almost dare not feel too much because then she will be totally exposed if things go wrong] and you don't know what the end result is going to feel like . . . yeah yeah that's probably why you know there's still a long road to travel and yeah its just so new. [I: and whether for some people I don't know really that's maybe a bit of a protective mechanism?] Yeah I was just thinking I was just wondering that that's probably why C is more he thinks everything will be fine and we'll go along fine and . . . [husband is situated as someone who is unable to be as insightful about the pregnancy] you know when we had our 12-week scan I noticed a big difference in me then from before it to after it you know things are alright' [reality of the baby conflicts with recognition that things may go wrong and to be pregnant and remain successfully pregnant]. [Mary_1_1]

The early thoughts here with regard to this excerpt of narrative were that Mary's failure to emotionally bond as much as she feels she should appear to be intimately connected with her fear that things may go wrong; she has accepted the responsibility of motherhood, unlike her husband who has engaged with the idealised fictional accounts and aspects of having a baby. Mary, in contrast has recognised the responsibility of parenthood from the very early stages of pregnancy.

Considering that one of the primary drivers of this research was to allow the previously subordinated voice of women to be heard, it felt important to continue to follow this intuitive feeling. One way of achieving this seemed to be to expand on this early approach to analysis. The concept that one actor can perform more than one role remained important but there was still a need to find a way of revealing the unarticulated narrative. The final method applied here to access the suppressed and unarticulated aspect of the narrative followed the work of Rogers, Casey, Ekert et al.[4]

LANGUAGES OF THE UNSAYABLE

Rogers and colleagues discuss the potential inherent in interpretivist poetics, which allows a reconceptualised approach to research analysis, reflecting the complexity of experience. They suggest that poetic images cannot be assigned to single categories without losing their multiple connotations and their capacity to evoke fresh responses every time they are encountered. This emphasis on variational images allows a useful model for approaching data, because we can acknowledge the presence of complex and multifaceted interpretation of narrative, drawing on the human capacity to hold multiple interpretations simultaneously. What is unsaid cannot be directly pinned down but the doublings of meaning that mark the dynamic interplay between the said and unsaid can be illustrated. They further suggest that the significance of what is present depends on what is absent, absent because it is too difficult or dangerous to articulate or because it simply cannot be expressed in the context of the interview. This presupposes that there is a range of other possibilities. From this frame what is said depends on what is not said for its full significance. Hence, this approach must systematically attend to what is said to 'define the landscape of the interview' but simultaneously be aware of the unsaid and the interplay between them. In this sense what is unsaid becomes a resource and a gateway for exploring the different layers of another person's encounters, experiences and understandings.[4] An example of how this worked within the women's stories might be salient here, utilising one narrative under the theme 'Change of status'.

> [E]rm . . . shock I think I don't know why because we had been trying for 9 months . . . I think you get to a point its almost as if you almost I, I'd suddenly gone into this phase where I thought I'm putting it out of my head now I'm not worrying about it so much and erm . . . I was getting used sort of not being pregnant every month and I think I was day later than the longest I'd ever been and I suddenly thought oh no now I'm going to be thinking oh dear am I am I am I better go and do a test just so I can and put it out of my head literally but erm but I didn't expect it to be positive erm shock and then I cried and ran round the house screaming my head off [laughs] really really pleased. [Mary_1_1]

The unsayable here seemed to be the inconceivable thought that Mary might never be pregnant. An underlying fear that she might never be a pregnant woman is not something that she feels able to articulate. She provides a smoke-screen response to this situation by suggesting that it's the worry that prevents her from becoming pregnant and if she stops worrying then it will happen. Society's emphasis on contraception makes women believe that getting pregnant is easy. So to accept that, despite trying, pregnancy was not happening for Mary is to acknowledge that she is unable to perform one of the primary functions expected of a woman. In this narrative there is simultaneously an attempt to reconcile not becoming pregnant with a desperate need to confirm the pregnancy. Her shock and excitement at the positive result of the pregnancy test, which creates the reality of pregnancy, is clearly narrated. When Mary recognises that she is now pregnant, two characters are created as she recognises that she is no longer the 'non-pregnant woman' of yesterday but the 'pregnant woman' of today. Yet the spectre of the 'non-pregnant woman' remains.

> '[A]lthough even within the first few months feeling so much better than I thought, I mean I can remember somebody I talked to and they said I must have that day felt a bit queasy or something and they turned round and said 'oh oh that's really really good' you know 'when you start to feel really sick it's a really really good sign because that means your pregnancy's all going you know your hormone levels are going up as they should be' and all this and like a few days after because I was feeling well again I was thinking I was thinking ooh . . . I know logically because I know people you know who have had good pregnancies as well which doesn't mean anything but that's the information you see cos I already knew that if I didn't know that I could be worrying about sort of . . .' [M_1_1]

There seems to be an underlying fear here of losing the baby or not actually being pregnant and returning to that non-pregnant state that existed prior to the positive pregnancy test and confirmation of the pregnant status.

REVEALING WOMEN'S IDENTITIES

Immersion in the data within the change of status theme, had resulted in the emergence of a suppressed voice that was that of the woman always preparing for pregnancy ('always pregnant women') and that of a woman waiting to be a mother ('mother in waiting'). These suppressed voices however, seemed to offer the way of accessing more than the singular identity and actions of pregnant women. In essence, they seemed to provide the key to reveal the hidden voices within the narratives, which all serve to comprise 'the narrative woman' and collectively construct her own personal and communal identity in pregnancy and childbirth. What clearly emerges within the following narratives is that 'the narrative woman' comprises more than one single voice.

What is apparent is that the actor (woman) can also be 'pregnant woman', 'mother', 'desired/undesired partner' all exposed by the narratives that she relates either explicitly or implicitly. Each woman consists of a number of identities, which are part of what makes them 'what/who they are'; these identities in turn are invested of their characteristics by the matrix of influences that surround them. The women narrated their experiences but in doing so reveal identities that are brought into being by their emotional and physical responses to the influences within their social and cultural sphere of experience.

The influential elements that construct a woman's experience may not be immediately apparent in the direct actions of the actors but are present in their narratives. The woman as an actor is distinguished by an historical anchoring in name and time but represents a number of identities defined and created by the influences present within her experience. For example: the system tells women how to be good mothers right from the moment of conception/ confirmed pregnancy. Health professionals provide instruction in eating well, avoiding risky behaviours and responsible pregnancy. Women are not critical of this system but conform; it is necessary to access the system to validate their pregnancy and confirm their new identity (pregnant woman). In addition, adopting the recommended behaviours confirms their identity within the collective 'pregnant woman' but also presents them as 'good pregnant woman' who adopts responsible behaviours in order to assure the well-being of her baby. Their narratives are an effect of the meaning and values in current circulation.

It is evident that others had roles to play within the narratives. Many of these, however, serve to consolidate the women's identities. The GP is a clear character within the early narratives but potentially performs several influencing roles, one of which is the role of validating the pregnancy and being the gatekeeper to the process and the system that recognises the woman as 'pregnant woman'. The pregnancy test, visiting the GP and accessing antenatal care all signify 'pregnant' and bring with them certain properties of a collective identity that is pregnant woman/mother.

Hence, the women here are being represented as sitting at the centre of an orbiting structure of influences some implicit and some explicit, which in turn will influence the woman and create the multiplicity of identities that constitute her. The identities within each narrative are in a sense shaped by one or more influences within the orbiting universe. The influences become apparent through the identities and in turn reveal the discourses and stimuli, which serve to construct women's contemporary maternity experience.

It seems clear that pregnant women require the maternity system, but as part of that system they are not enabled to have a voice – it is unacceptable to step outside that frame. Their articulated stories are constrained by the frame of the interview and their current status, and only allow them to articulate, firstly, the things associated with pregnancy/motherhood and, secondly, the acceptable discourses of their maternity experience. What this model for analysis has enabled is both an identification of the unspoken voices and a way of accessing women's multiple voices/identities within the text, as well as how those multiple identities are created and what discourses/influences bring about their creation. It also identifies how women construct and experience pregnancy, birth and motherhood in the way that they do. What discourses, advice and influences do they accept and which do they reject? And what informs both this acceptance and rejection? Such an approach has created an illuminating account of women's physical and emotional maternity experience but also the influences and discourses that inform their choices and decisions during this time.

SUMMARY

This chapter has briefly outlined the emergent and reflexive approach employed in the analysis of women's stories. One aim has been to ensure a transparency in the analytical frameworks development, which promotes confidence in the interpretations to follow in Chapters 5 to 8. Chapters 5 and 6 will present interpretations of the women's antenatal accounts in both early and late pregnancy. Chapters 7 and 8 will focus on the postnatal accounts, which were obtained at 14 days and six months following the birth of the women's babies.

The following chapters present the narrative themes identified in the interviews undertaken, and through the application of the analytical framework the narrative influences and identities present within those themes. Themes, which appeared in the narratives of all the women, will be identified and discussed. One interviewee's account was unfortunately abandoned due to the poor quality of the recordings. In order to assist in the presentation of a coherent narrative, which is difficult given the number of interviews and the amount of data gathered, the themes will be illustrated and discussed throughout using the narratives of two key participants.[2] Excerpts from the other interviews are used to demonstrate not only that the recurrent themes in each participant's story are reflected in other women's narratives, but also to develop understanding of the 'choice in childbirth' narratives. The focus is upon Mary and Helen, chosen because of their differing profiles and preferences for place of delivery. What is shown is both how individual and unique each woman's story is, and, strikingly, how each is influenced by many similar underlying influences. The following chapters expose the narrative identities that the social and cultural influences construct within the women's stories and reveal those influences within the women's narratives. To aid clarity, the influencing factors will be depicted in *italics* and the women's identities in **bold**.

It is important to emphasise that these interviews are with a specific group of women, with no known significant medical or obstetric problems when recruited, and so suitable for choice within maternity care. In addition they were all motivated and able to access all available maternity care. It must be acknowledged that there are many other women whose circumstances in pregnancy are more personally or medically adverse and as such would not be seen at booking to be suitable for choice.

Brief pen portraits of all the women are presented to provide background information. Pseudonyms are used throughout to protect the women's anonymity.

Mary: A 31-year-old nurse, married to Matt with her own home, and pregnant for the first time with a planned pregnancy after a period of trying; delighted to be pregnant. Mary is surrounded by a local network of family and friends.

Helen: A 36-year-old housewife and mother, with a stable partner but unmarried. Living in local authority housing, she already has two girls, one 11-year-old from a previous relationship and one four-year-old to her current partner Phil. Pregnant for the third time with an unplanned pregnancy and initially unhappy with the situation, Helen has very little in terms of family support, as her own family do not live locally.

Sally: A 33-year-old with a full time career, married to John, they own their own home. Sally is pregnant for the first time; although the pregnancy was planned she appears ambivalent about being pregnant. Sally has family living nearby and lots of friends, although many do not live local to her.

Polly: A 38-year-old, full-time account manager, married to James with their own home. Delighted to be pregnant for the first time, with a planned pregnancy, after trying for a number of months and feeling anxious about not conceiving. Polly does not have family living nearby but her family are extremely supportive. She is surrounded by a network of friends.

Julie: A 36-year-old, married for the second time to Rob, with a 13-year-old daughter from her first marriage. Pregnant after IVF treatment, with a much-wanted pregnancy, Julie and Rob are delighted to be pregnant. Julie owns her own home and works part-time. Julie has a strong local network of family and friends.

Jane: A 30-year-old, married to Paul. They are a professional couple who own their home. This was a planned pregnancy and Jane is pleased to be pregnant. Jane works full-time and intends to return to work after having had her baby. Jane has both family and friends living locally.

Jan: A 40-year-old, married to Scott, they already have two children, a boy aged seven and girl aged ten. They own their own home. Pregnant with an unplanned pregnancy, Jan was initially shocked to be pregnant but is now pleased. Jan works part-time at the local hospital as an administrator. Jan is surrounded by a local network of family and friends.

Kate: A 21-year-old, single mother of a two-year-old. Living in local authority housing, she has a current partner but he does not live with her and is not currently living in the same geographic area. Kate did not plan her pregnancy and initially was not pleased to be pregnant. Kate receives a lot of support from her family and has a local network of friends. She is not currently working.

Sophie: A 26-year-old receptionist, married to Karl, with a three-year-old. They own their own home. Pregnant for the second time with a planned pregnancy, Sophie is happy to be pregnant. Sophie has good family support and a local group of friends.

REFERENCES

1 Murray M. Narrative psychology. In: Smith JA, editor. *Qualitative Psychology*. London: Sage; 2003.

2 Hollway W, Jefferson T. *Doing Qualitative Research Differently*. 3rd ed. London: Sage; 2000.

3 Sunderland J. *Gendered Discourses*. Basingstoke: Palgrave Macmillan; 2004.

4 Rogers AG, Casey ME, Ekert J, *et al*. An interpretive poetics of languages of the unsayable. In: Josselson R, Leiblich A, editors. *Making Meaning of Narratives*. Thousand Oaks, CA: Sage; 1999.

5 Crotty M. *The Foundations of Social Research: meaning and perspective in the research process*. London: Sage; 1998.

6 Czarniawska B. *Narratives in Social Science Research*. London: Sage; 2004.

7 Greimas AJ. *Structural Semantics: an attempt at method*. Schleifer R, McDowell D, trans. Lincoln: University of Nebraska Press; 1983.

8 Greimas AJ, Courtes J. *Semiotics and Language: an analytical dictionary*. Crist L, Patte D, Lee J, McMahon E, Philips G, Rangstorf F, trans. Bloomington: Indiana University Press; 1982.

9 Belsey C. *Poststructuralism: a very short introduction*. New York: Oxford University Press; 2002.

CHAPTER 5

Now I'm pregnant: early pregnancy and choices for care

12–14 WEEKS PREGNANT

The following section presents women's early (12–14 weeks) pregnancy experiences. The themes identified here were common across all interviews and establish much of the context for women's maternity experience as a whole. These early themes include:

- a new identity
- physical pregnancy
- the new identity, ownership and choice
- the GP gatekeeper
- the new identity, naturalness, responsibility and emotions
- promoting motherhood/relegating fatherhood
- perfect babies and screening choice
- experts and expertise.

A NEW IDENTITY

The result of a *pregnancy test* creates a change of status from that of **non-pregnant woman** to **pregnant woman,** and it seems that some kind of transition begins at this stage. The *pregnancy test* therefore emerges as influential very early within the narratives. Mary here shows that although previously pregnancy tests had confirmed that she was non-pregnant, there had always been a sense of expectation. By the time of the interview she is no longer a **non-pregnant woman** but a **pregnant woman.** This recognition that she is no longer what she was prior to the *pregnancy test* is both shocking and exciting.

> [E]rm . . . shock I think I don't know why because we had been trying for 9 months . . . I was getting used [to] sort of not being pregnant every month and I think I was a day later than the longest I'd ever been and I suddenly thought oh no now I'm going to be thinking oh dear am I am I am I, I better go and do a test just so I can and put it out of my head literally but erm but I didn't expect it to be positive, erm shock and then I cried and ran round the house screaming my head off [laughs] really really pleased. [Mary_1_3]

The *pregnancy test* result, which was discussed by all interviewees, appears to play an integral role in the shift from non-pregnant to pregnant woman. This can be seen in Helen's account. Having been pregnant twice before, *personal knowing*, meaning an innate sense of her own body, leads her to suspect that she is pregnant. However, the *pregnancy test* is still necessary to confirm her as a **pregnant woman**.

> I did a home testing kit, I **knew** before I'd even missed a period sort of and he said 'well you can't be' and I said 'I know that I'm pregnant' so before I'd even missed a period I knew that I was pregnant, cos I'd had the same sort of sickness before even before I'd missed a period I'd had a few days of not feeling too well. I said 'I think I'm pregnant', he said 'Well you haven't even missed a period', and I said 'I don't need to I know I'm gonna be late'. A few days passed and I thought 'I haven't started' so I did a kit and it came back positive and I took one into the doctors about a week later. [Helen_1_2]

Kate similarly relates how, despite previous experience of pregnancy, *personal knowing* is insufficient, again highlighting the importance to women of the *pregnancy test* result in confirming them as '**pregnant woman**'.

> I don't know because I never had regular periods anyway [I: right] erm I think it was just the fact that my boobs felt heavy and that's what I kind of had when I was expecting this one so I just thought I might be pregnant. I did one test er a couple of weeks before hand and it said I wasn't and then I did one a couple of weeks later and it said I was so . . . I was a bit like am I or aren't I but then I went for my scan and I wasn't as far on as I thought I was, I was only 8 weeks where as I thought I was actually 12. [Kate_1_1]

Mary's story tells that both she and her partner are ready for new roles (motherhood/fatherhood). The transition to the role in a planned pregnancy begins with the decision to have a baby, but the reality of the situation is only provided by the concrete evidence of the positive *pregnancy test*. Initial delight at the positive result is replaced by concerns about the reality and responsibilities of this new parenting role.

> [S]uddenly you realise you're in this for nine months and you have to face things . . . were ready for a new chapter in our lives we were ready for that [I: mm mm] but then wanting it and then having it are two different things aren't they [I: mm] so you've still got that adjustment to make haven't you? [Mary_1_3]

Jan's account also supports the importance of the *pregnancy test* in constructing the **pregnant woman**. When the result is positive, the recognition that things are different occurs immediately.

> [A]nd they're all saying you know 'go to the toilets and do one now . . . do it now' and I said 'oh it'll be negative I've you know I've just got PMT bit longer than usual' I couldn't believe it . . . but I went white apparently as I came out I was as white as a sheet . . . [I: So how did you feel about being pregnant then?] Erm . . . disbelief really at first but I was really happy . . . I felt a bit numb to be honest, [I: mm] my third pregnancy, I thought I'm a bit older and to balance two children with working and the house and that I thought 'oh crikey how will I cope' but erm I was happy . . . I couldn't believe it yet I was shocked with my other two I think even if you plan pregnancy its still a big shock [I: mm I think you're right] when it happens and those lines appear. [Jan_1_1]

The confirmed presence of a fetus via the *pregnancy test* creates an identity that did not exist before. What becomes apparent is that recognition of themselves as **pregnant women** means that women now situate the fetus as a significant influence. For example, Mary above suggests that having a baby is both the start of a new chapter and something more than that, i.e. the acceptance of a responsibility implicit in parenthood. The presence of the fetus demands of both Mary and her partner that they become something new, taking on a role that hasn't existed for them before the pregnancy.

Helen's feelings about her pregnancy are less positive, but it also leads to the realisation that she is different to before and that there are associated implications.

> I wasn't at first, it wasn't planned I mean I was taking the pill and it was a total out of the blue shock it was you know we didn't want any more, got two so you know sort of huge shock to the system really . . . No, no we did sort of think well should I go ahead with it or shouldn't I you know we had 2 or 3 days where we both sat thinking mm don't think we can afford it, we haven't got

no room, next thing was I think we could probably manage and then it was we can't manage, we can manage, we can't manage and we spent a whole 2 days, one minute we was having it then we weren't, we were, we weren't, we were, we weren't . . . I think if now like obviously I'm 15 weeks not I think if I'd have looked back and thought well decided not to keep it I think it probably would have haunted me I think well come next year when it would have been due I'd have probably regretted it. [Helen_1_2]

In all these accounts the influence of the *fetus* via the *pregnancy test* in achieving the transition to **pregnant woman** is clear. What is also apparent in Helen's narrative is that once the presence of the *fetus* is confirmed it plays a significant role ('it probably would have haunted me') in decisions to maintain the pregnancy. Helen's unplanned pregnancy demonstrates that the repositioning from **non-pregnant woman** to **pregnant woman** may be difficult or unwelcome.

The active role women ascribe to the *fetus* is supported by the apparent emotional connection and inherent responsibility women discuss in relation to the fetus. In Helen's description of making the right decision, where to terminate would be a wrong decision, the influential role of the fetus is demonstrated through its having a potential that will be prevented if it is not allowed to become a baby. This sentiment about terminations is clearly echoed by Kate.

I wasn't happy but . . . it's on its way now I don't agree with terminations. [Kate_1_1]

The above narratives show that women experience a new identity from early in pregnancy. The transition to this new identity is affected by the desire, or not, to be pregnant, but is reinforced by the confirmed existence of the *fetus* and early feelings of responsibility and attachment that women display with regard to the *fetus*.

PHYSICAL PREGNANCY

It seems that concurrent with this new identity of **pregnant woman** is the importance of physical symptoms in the normality of this new identity. The *fetus* causes physiological changes that allow confirmation of the pregnancy by the *pregnancy test*, and create the **pregnant woman** identity. In addition, its presence is believed to cause a bodily response in symptoms such as nausea and vomiting, which are associated with *cultural recognition of the pregnant state*.[1,2] Mary's narrative shows that physical symptoms are a visible and accepted way of reinforcing the **normal pregnant woman** identity. The absence of feeling ill in early pregnancy is a source of anxiety that she is an **abnormal pregnant woman**.

> I can remember somebody I talked to and they said I must have that day felt a bit queasy or something and they turned round and said 'oh oh that's really really good' you know 'when you start to feel really sick it's a really really good sign because that means your pregnancy all going you know your hormone levels are going up as they should be' and all this and like a few days after because I was feeling well again I was thinking I was thinking ooh . . . I know logically because I know people you know who have had good pregnancies as well which doesn't mean anything but that's the information you see cos I already knew that if I didn't know that I could be worrying about sort of. [Mary_1_3]

This sentiment was echoed by Polly.

> I haven't had any effects that you should normally get like the morning sickness, tiredness, erm, anything like that its been very very straight forward to the point where I've not really believed that I am. [Polly_1_1]

That physical symptoms should approximate to some norm is shown from the other extreme by Helen. She suffers all the expected physical symptoms and is concerned that, as they extend beyond the expected period of time, they are not consistent with *western depictions of pregnancy*. She is therefore an **abnormal pregnant woman** who is concerned that her symptoms will impact on the wellbeing of the baby. This is implicit in the suggestion that she will feel reassured after having a *scan*, which plays an important role in confirming her baby as normal and healthy.

> **Horrible,** sickness, all the usual, headache . . . not feeling too well at all . . . It did go it did sort of 7–12 weeks I was really violently ill all day long couldn't eat anything drink anything and it stopped I thought yes I was eating alright for 2 weeks and its come back again headache, heartburn so if I do have a nice meal I get really bad heartburn so I'm eating these anti-acid things like sweets and so I can't win got blinding headache its . . . I think. I've been suffering for about 3 months I think I'll feel a bit better when I've been for my scan and I've sort of seen it. [Helen_1_2]

Other women's accounts narrate a pattern that is concordant with the *western depictions of pregnancy*, where nausea and vomiting are a temporary state. Women show that there is a norm in these depictions by which they judge their perform-ance as **normal pregnant women**.

> Fine . . . the first 12 weeks I just felt tired and crappy and sickly, I wasn't actually sick I just felt very very sick and then I felt a lot better. [Sally_1_1]

> [A] bit more sick a lot more nausea I haven't actually been sick but erm I've been off my food a bit but its come back with a vengeance my appetite now for about 4 or 5 weeks. [Jan_1_1]

It can therefore be seen that *western depictions of pregnancy* has a significant role in women's expectations of their physical experience in early pregnancy and in reinforcing their identity of **normal pregnant woman**. The significance of this is the apparent anxiety provoked in women; that they are an **abnormal pregnant woman** if their experiences do not entirely concord with those depictions

A further influential discourse in the narratives above for both Mary and Helen is that of *cultural ideas about what women represent in society*. Despite feminist challenges and the changing demographics with regard to working mothers, social attitudes and policies continue to lag behind.[3] A woman's role for many remains institutionalised; women have a clear and distinct role, which fundamentally involves producing normal healthy children. Although informed by completely different experiences, both Mary and Helen's narra-tives suggest a fear of being an **abnormal pregnant woman**, which suggests a failure in adequately performing one of women's essential life roles as defined by cultural ideas about womanhood. This cultural expectation is a powerful socialising force that defines a restricted range of options within which women's individual pregnancy experience is located. All these discourses are located within a pronatalist society. Infertility or lack of ability to carry a pregnancy to a successful conclusion creates a crisis for women in fulfilling their social role. It seems reasonable then to claim that the perfusion of these discourses can be identified in the way that despite the distinctively unique experience for each woman of being pregnant, they each demonstrate how similar these influences are within each account.

THE NEW IDENTITY, OWNERSHIP AND CHOICE

The positive pregnancy test has created a new **pregnant woman**. The existence of the *fetus* is now a reality that brings with it responsibilities. In these early interviews the woman sets the scene and develops her role as the integral/central character in the story. What also emerges in these accounts of early pregnancy is women's ownership of their pregnancies; by 'ownership' I mean 'her property'. Pregnancy is located as a physical event that is happening to her and which excludes her partner. Mary's partner had been clearly involved in the decision to try for a baby and Helen's partner had been similarly involved in the consideration of a termination. However, as these women recount the progression of their pregnancies, partners are excluded from their accounts. It seems that even if women initially refer to the pregnancy as jointly owned, they proceed to take ownership of the pregnancy and the decisions associated with it. Decision-making is accepted as a personal responsibility. This can be seen in their repeated use of the pronoun 'I' and use of the first person, suggesting that women regard their pregnancies as a personalised rather than a dualised event, and in doing so choices and decisions are made within that context of individual ownership. If pregnancy were perceived as a shared experience we would expect recurring references to 'we' and 'our' within these early narratives. Although there are some uses of the plural, slippage clearly occurs and what begins as a plural experience changes largely to a singular one. This can be illustrated through the ways in which advice is taken from *experts*, either in the form of informed friends or professionals, who are perceived as being in touch with women's feelings and concerns. Mary's account illustrates this.

> [I]t was talking to friends erm . . . a couple of people had said really nice things about Mr X, having said that I feel felt very relaxed about being pregnant I wasn't I knew that the tests that you go for were standard . . . and I have a lot of confidence in midwives so . . . having sort of though all of that and also talking it all over at that first check . . . I have a check up with a midwife every time . . . [I: so you didn't feel you needed that consultant input antenatally?] No [I: but you felt you wanted to deliver at the consultant unit?] yessss . . . erm I suppose I mean as times going on its erm I sort of wonder you see I know the birth centre they don't its just midwifery led [I: yes] and as times going on I feel more confident that that would have been alright but with it everything being such a first for me you know I know that if anything happens or interpret expressions on peoples faces during labour the wrong way I will start getting worried about it that I would feel happier being in somewhere if things go wrong then they can do something about it quickly. [Mary_1_3]

This is mirrored in Polly's account.

> I went to see the doctor and she sat down and explained you know . . . then asked me to make a decision of which hospital I wanted to go to . . . That's how I made the decision. [Polly_1_1]

Interestingly, there is no questioning of the necessity of input from healthcare professionals during pregnancy. Mary's account shows that she makes her decisions for antenatal care based on convenience to her, but also shows how in early pregnancy women feel that the normality of a pregnancy can only be judged in retrospect, i.e. after the pregnancy is completed. This is part of the acknowledged *medical discourse* that surrounds maternity care,[4] and what is important for this analysis is the influential role *the medical discourse* plays in informing Mary's decisions and her presentation of herself as a **responsible pregnant woman** (e.g. 'I would feel happier being in somewhere if things go wrong then they can do something about it quickly'). Her choices are then made within that context out of a belief that this is the best way to ensure her pregnancy ends with a live, healthy baby. Kate's and Sally's responses to choice of place for delivery also show how *the medical discourse* influences in promoting them as **responsible pregnant woman** and the underpinning rationale of their accounts mirrors Mary's.

> Well I chose to go to the Royal because . . . if I did have any problems, I wouldn't want to lose the baby. [Kate_1_1]

> I'd rather be in a hospital where there's everything I need so that would no, it wouldn't have made any difference and if they had told me then I wouldn't have taken all the information in you can't take everything in so I think it's been fine. [Sally_1_1]

Polly's account similarly reflects the influence of *the medical discourse*. Although proximity and ease of access is an important consideration for some women when making choices for delivery, these do not supersede the ultimate well-being of the baby. Decisions are made based on ensuring the best care provision for their babies should problems arise, and it is '*the medical discourse*' that informs how these decisions are considered.

> I went to see the doctor and she sat down and explained all the, you know, all the availability of care in the area and then asked me to make a decision of which hospital I wanted to go to. I think she gave me a choice of three . . . for me I felt that one was nearer although I did ask the question obviously if any of them had better care than the others and she said 'no all three were generally the same' erm one was probably more specialised and therefore if there were any problems at all then myself and the baby would probably be transferred to one of them during labour and that's how I made the decision. [Polly_1_1]

Helen's story demonstrates the slightly different way in which the *medical discourse* continues to pervade the contemporary model of choice for maternity care. Her narrative is reported in some length here, as it illustrates well the significant and transformative influence of *medical discourse* on her narrative identity. She begins with recounting a visit to her GP.

> [H]e sort of just said 'what type of birth did you want?' and I said I would have liked a home birth 'I don't agree with home births' and that was his [answer] 'I don't agree with home births and erm I think you should go to . . .' and I said well I would really like a home birth purely for I wouldn't have to try and sort the kids out but no he didn't agree with a home birth and he basically said 'I don't agree with a home birth I think you should go here blah blah blah' but when you go to the booking in clinic discuss it with them basically that was it, that was all he said, but he didn't really agree with a home birth and he didn't even agree with then birth centre . . . he's all for the new hospital [I: So what did he say then about them then?] Yeah he said he didn't agree with the . . . birth centre purely because it was run by midwives, there's no doctors or obstetricians there and he thinks that by having your baby there if anything goes wrong you're then putting not just my life in danger but the baby's life as well . . . so he thinks I should go straight to the new one, but from our point of view the birth centre's just up the road. [I: So did his opinions influence your choice in any way?] Well I thought 'have I got a choice?' I went to the booking in clinic and said 'well judging by the doctor I haven't got a choice' and he basically said 'he doesn't want me to have a home birth, he doesn't agree with it, he doesn't agree with the birth centre' the only choice then is the new one. I spoke to the midwife at the booking-in clinic and she said you can go where you want basically, so I've booked in for the birth centre and then she rung me back to say that I'd been told to go to the new one if I go before 38 weeks. [I: So what made you choose the birth centre, I know you've already said it's easier and nearer but are there any other reasons you would want to deliver there rather than at the main maternity unit?] Erm . . . well for one it's nearer and two I've had two straightforward births with no complications they've both been very quick so from that point of view I just couldn't have gone there. [Helen_1_2]

Helen's story demonstrates the numerous issues surrounding choice. On first reading, it could be construed that Helen is an **irresponsible pregnant woman** basing her choices on ease and access, rather than the well-being of her baby. Her rationale for her choice, however, is more complex. It involves the influence of *personal knowing*. Her two previous early but unproblematic births make her feel no need for the support of that medical intervention, which Mary, as a first-time mother, feels is necessary. Helen's previous experience within the frame of *expert knowing* does, however, limit her choice, because she does not entirely fit within the medically defined frame of normality. Her choice, being that of a **responsible pregnant woman** as defined by *medical discourse*, is made, like Mary's, with the well-being of her baby in mind. The precipitant nature of her previous deliveries generates concerns that she might not actually reach the main hospital. Therefore, delivering at the birth centre or by home birth assures the presence of an *expert* in case any problems should arise. This interpretation is supported in her account of her last delivery.

> Oh yeah I know that if it comes before 38 weeks then the new hospitals got to be the best place to have my baby regardless of whether I want to go there or not, I mean the main concern is getting to the new one with my second one she was extremely quick I mean we was living at Wxxx at the time and we had to travel to the hospital and I mean we got there at 8.30 on the Friday night and she was born at 8.35 on the Friday night, we literally just got through the doors, got on the bed and out she popped [I: right, right] . . . she sort of just popped out and that was it and poor Phil . . . so I really want to be somewhere close cos I think if I do go in I'm gonna you know . . . [I: you don't want an unplanned home birth] No, no. [Helen_1_2]

Jane refers to her choice to deliver at the birth centre. Her choice does not seem based predominantly on her baby's well-being but on considerations of personal anxieties and perceptions of the support she feels will be necessary in labour. The infusion of the medical model is less apparent in this narrative but delivery still relies on the presence of an *expert*, which in this case is the midwife. While Jane appears to be rejecting *the medical discourse* ('I hate needles'), she is still acting through the discourse of *expert*. Through choice Jane rejects the medical model but it remains intrinsic within her story.

> Because I hate needles and the thought of it just makes me feel . . . I'd rather have the pain. I don't know how I'm going to be with the pain but I'll just deal with it and Paul will be there and the midwife will be there to help me. [Jane_2_1]

Women have outlined choice here as extremely complex, based on consideration of a number of orbiting influences. The ultimate choice women make seems dependant on which of these influences they accept and which they reject. Within that claim however it needs to be acknowledged that the influences and discourse implicit in the women's narratives actually limit the possibilities of choice. In her new identity as firstly **pregnant woman** and then **responsible**

pregnant woman, the woman takes ownership of the pregnancy from her partner. That ownership then appears to be ceded to the medical/midwifery professions, because of the dominance of culturally-accepted knowledge that expertise is the best way of ensuring a successful birth outcome. Quality of care is important but in the main remains secondary to their baby's well-being. Even women such as Jane who choose the birth centre for delivery are still ensuring the presence of an *expert*, and so are not entirely rejecting 'a medical model'. The *consumerist discourse of choice* does seem to offer the possibility of resistance to 'the medical discourse' even if it does not fundamentally question the necessity of expertise or remains unfulfilled. Helen epitomises this unfulfilled resistance and how she feels that she has no real choice. Helen's narrative around choice afforded a clear role to the GP, and it is therefore important that the GP is individually considered as part of *the medical discourse* that, even in a changing climate of maternity care, often demands he is accessed as part of pregnancy.

THE GP GATEKEEPER

The GP is an unmistakable and influential character who appears to hold a powerful position within the women's early pregnancy experiences. All the women define him/her as the first point of contact following the positive *pregnancy test*.

> Erm . . . rang my GP I think yeah . . . I wasn't I wasn't sure cos I mean I really made an appointment and went to see him and he said 'oh yeah fine' they don't do they don't bother testing you now do they, [I: no] come back in a few more weeks when you're a bit further along and . . . yes he gave me some do and don'ts . . . he sort of outlined really whatever I wanted to do and it was fine. [Mary_1_3]

The importance of the GP being the first point of contact is illustrated in Jan's narrative, which suggests that visiting the GP is a step in a process, because the *GP expert*, as a medical expert, plays a role in further validating the pregnancy that has been confirmed by the *pregnancy test*. He acts as a *GP gatekeeper*, opening the doorway to the maternity system, which ratifies the pregnancy and further confirms her as a **pregnant woman**.

> I contacted my doctors and asked if I could pop in real early in the morning on the way to work, to get erm . . . you know one of those a urine test bottle thing [I: mm] and I had to hand that it so that you know I'd know for definite, I think he likes you to do that my GP here, then its confirmed and it really hits home

as well doesn't it? I mean I know those tests are 99% that are in shops but that's a 100% that one [laughs] so that was the next step. [Jan_1_1]

The GP's role as a *GP expert* and a *GP gatekeeper* is supported in Sally's account.

> [S]o then I did a test and I thought that looks positive I'll do another test and show it to John and he was like 'well it looks positive to me' so we went to the doctors and I said 'I think I am I've done two tests . . . and he said that we were and confirmed it for definite [I: right] . . . I went back again . . . to the doctors and he said that it was all confirmed and that everything had been okay and he referred me at that point. [Sally_1_1]

The role of the *GP gatekeeper* lies in defining or not defining the woman as **normal pregnant woman** and thus eligible to make choices. One of the ways in which the GP does this is through the amount and content of the advice proffered. Mary was offered an explanation of the options for care and place of delivery and given an opportunity to consider them. Her *GP expert* situates her as a **normal pregnant woman** who fits the criteria for choice. For Helen, however, despite local service reconfiguration, her *GP expert* acts as a barrier to choice. Acting as the mouthpiece for *medical discourse* he removed all sense of choice from Helen at her first visit, thus preventing her from being a **normal pregnant woman**. The main blame for Helen's perceived lack of choice can be attributed to the GP, however, the midwife also only offers limited choices.[5] In Helen's case she is only able to access a home birth or midwifery-led care if she can redefine herself as a **normal pregnant woman**, which glosses over how normal comes to be socially, culturally and historically defined. She describes the *GP gatekeeper/expert* as having won, suggesting that choice is a battle. Situating Helen as an **abnormal pregnant woman** renders her powerless to enforce her own choice, because as a responsible pregnant woman she is unprepared to challenge expertise.

> I sort of got the impression from what he said that if I decided I was going to have a home birth then he sort of said I wouldn't want to deal with the pregnancy so from my point of view he was trying to say to me if you choose to have a home birth then I don't want you at my antenatal you'll go through another doctor but I mean from that point of view I think its won, in a way you don't feel you've got a choice I don't think, it's a case of well the doctor's said no, the midwife said no I'll have to have a baby where they say [I: yeah] so when she said I was having it at the birth centre I thought oh that's fine but then she said

unless you go to 38 weeks you're going to the new one so I thought, I was a bit, I was a bit gutted. [Helen_1_2]

Jan's narrative suggests a similar experience in the referral that the *GP gatekeeper* makes without any real discussion. She has been labeled abnormal due to her previous experience and her age, despite a normal delivery with her daughter.

[B]ut I've not been very pleased with what my doctor been saying to me actually. [I: in what way] Erm . . . I sat down today and he said 'so you're pregnant again' and I said 'a bit of a surprise' like this and he said 'what didn't work . . . I would have thought at your age you'd know about contraception' he wasn't joking; I thought 'oh' I just felt like walking out I couldn't believe it, so . . . that's the attitude really that's what I got . . . I said 'I realize at my age I'll have to have well I don't have to but I'll be offered extra tests and things and it might come back high risk or whatever' and he said 'of course it will at your **age**' . . . that's made me a bit paranoid I know I'm not a spring chicken . . . but I'm not the oldest mother in the world either. [Jan_1_1]

The *GP expert* here, again plays a significant role, acts as the mouthpiece of a *medical discourse* that positions older women as at-risk, and creates a fear and anxiety in Jan that wasn't present before her visit to him. In positioning her as an **abnormal pregnant woman**, he refers her without any discussion about options for care, despite the fact she would not have been excluded from midwifery-led care options. Jan's identity as a **responsible pregnant woman** makes her, despite her annoyance, complicit in accepting this referral as the best thing and justifies it as the option she would have chosen.

Erm . . . yes he said were you under a consultant when you had Sam because he knew he had intrauterine growth retardation, I wasn't with that GP at the time [I: right] when I had Sam, so I said yes Mr Z so he said right I'm going to write to him . . . I was thinking blimey hurry up I want to know what's going on . . . I was actually pleased with that anyway, Mr Z cos I used to work next door to the women's and children's health anyway and he used to wave to me in the canteen I quite liked Mr Z [laughs]. I would have approached my GP and said could I do that with my history. [Jan_1_1]

The GP is both a character within the story but also as an influence through his unspoken role as *GP gatekeeper* and *GP expert*, which constructs women as **normal pregnant women** or **abnormal pregnant women** at almost the earliest point in their pregnancies. This powerful role of GPs as, most often, the women's first point of contact can clearly create difficulties in offering women choices for care. Indeed, these narratives would suggest that choice for some women is as difficult to achieve now as it was in the 1980s when authors like Oakley described lack of choice and control in pregnancy and childbirth.[6] The actantial role of the *GP expert* in defining women as 'normal' or 'abnormal' suggests they are gatekeeping in a way different from anticipated, making decisions about who is suitable for the gate marked 'choice'. For those marked 'abnormal', their identity as a **responsible pregnant woman** encourages complicity in the refusal of choice.

THE NEW IDENTITY, NATURALNESS, RESPONSIBILITY AND EMOTIONS

Mary and Helen exemplify the women in this study in their articulation of a clear acceptance of the responsibility inherent in being pregnant. Texts around pregnancy and the maternity care system construct pregnant women as made whole, as a vessel or incubator for the baby.[5] Their role, therefore, is one of nurturance and protection, the providers of the environment for the fetus and as such responsible for their baby's health.[4] The most relevant ideological discourse here is the naturalness of practices associated with 'mothering'. Althusser, discussed in Sunderland, refers to naturalness as something imposed but without the appearance of imposition.[7] The naturalness discourses of the women's narratives are located within natural gendered parenting discourses. *Cultural representations of mothers* frequently idealise motherhood and prescribe what 'good mothers' do and how they should behave,[5] and the above discussion has shown how this even penetrates to how they regard their morning sickness during pregnancy. This provides a framework for society and women themselves to evaluate the behaviour of women as mothers. Where previous accounts locate the naturalness of mothering late in pregnancy or following the birth,[5] what is striking in these accounts is that women are aspiring and displaying this naturalness of mothering in early pregnancy, demonstrating feelings of nurturance and caring traditionally associated with good mothering after the birth. Mary, for example, narrates about adhering to advised behaviours promoting herself as a **good mother**, nurturing and protecting her baby.

> I'm making sure I do everything right I try and sort of do the right things. [Mary_1_3]

Similarly Polly and Kate narrate **good mother** behaviours.

[A]s long as I'm feeling well and I'm trying to do the right thing by eating by having a healthy diet and staying off the alcohol and all of those and maybe exercising its to me that's the right way to go. [Polly _1_1

I made an appointment at the doctors because I knew I needed folic acid anyway, so I went to see them to get some folic acid. [Kate_1_1]

What is interesting as Mary's narrative continues is that ensuring the well-being of the baby is both a physical and emotional act. The emotional aspects of Mary's narrative take a dichotomous format; the emotional relationship with the baby, which she refers to below and the personal psychological/emotional impact of pregnancy on her, which will be discussed later in this section.

I suppose that's something else I thought I'd feel more attached than I do I guess . . . I'm talking to it and I'm trying to imagine he or she as a person and erm this kind of thing [I: mm mm] . . . you see I thought when I first started to feel it move I thought I'd be absolutely overwhelmed with this that's my **baby** you know and it hasn't been quite that intense . . . but I think that will maybe come more gradually for me. [Mary_1_3]

This naturalness of mothering that involves an emotional invisible bond with the child seems to be influential in shaping Mary's own views of motherhood and expectations in pregnancy. Mary's first narrative expresses a sense of guilt that her feelings towards her baby are not as strong as they should be. This suggests the need to adhere to some kind of *cultural standard of bonding*. Bonding and maternal instincts are accepted concepts that are socially reinforced[5] and influentially act here by creating an expectation in Mary that this emotional bond should be an instinctive rather than learnt emotion. Mary throughout her narratives has presented herself as a **good mother**, evident in her physical actions, but also in a clear attachment to her fetus, which has motivated her to act appropriately and make responsible decisions. Inadequate mothers conversely are characterised by a lack of sufficient care, positive emotion, knowledge, insight and action.[8] Despite Mary's successful fulfilment of these characteristics, she questions her ability to attain this *cultural standard of bonding* and make an emotional connection to her baby; she considers the inability to do this as a failure. In an attempt to promote a feeling of bonding Mary tries to imagine her baby and attribute it with characteristics and a personality, but for her the baby remains unknown and intangible. This culturally mediated expectation creates conflict for Mary between two identities, the **good mother** who is acting responsibly in her behaviours and the **bad mother** who is unable to form a significant relationship or emotional bond with her baby.

The *scan* again acts as an important influence. Whilst it earlier served to confirm for some women their **pregnant woman** status, it now provides confirmation of them as **good mothers**. This provides *expert* reassurance that through their efforts to behave appropriately and responsibly, the pregnancy is progressing normally and the baby is healthy.

> [Y]ou know when we had our 12-week scan I noticed a big difference in me then from before it to after it you know things are alright. [Mary_1_3]

Polly also attaches importance to the *scan* to confirm normality.

> Obviously I've had an initial scan to put my mind at rest I think there is always that erm . . . there's always that concern in the back of your mind is everything going to be okay but obviously from what I've read they can't really tell you a great deal from this 14-week scan its more your 20-week scan where they go into it, into the pregnancy in more depth . . . but for me its more to put my mind at rest that everything is progressing as it should be and everything is growing as it should be and everything's in place. [Polly_1_1]

Sally expresses the ability of the scan to reveal abnormality as well as normality. The pictures she receives depict a normal healthy fetus and so reassure her that she is both a **normal pregnant woman** and a **good mother** because everything is normal.

> Fine yeah yeah fine I've got some pictures of it so that's okay [I: Were you looking forward to it?] . . . A bit nervous cos I mean they're checking more and things like that so a bit nervous. [Sally_1_1]

For Helen knowledge of the sex is additionally important, with some suggestion that this might promote an emotional connection, although this is quickly countered by Helen's **good mother** identity, which suggests that it is the normality and health of the baby that is a priority.

> Yeah, my scan's 4 weeks on Friday [I: right, are you looking forward to that] I am yeah, yeah basically to find out what it is [I: you want to know] oh yeah I do yeah [I: do you mind] . . . Erh, I'd like a boy because we've already got two girls and I know he'd like a boy as well but you get what you're given [I: you do] as

long as its all there and its healthy it doesn't really matter but its going to be the last one definite, so you know I'd like it to be a boy, both his sisters have got all the boys [I: right] and I've got all the girls so [I: it would be nice though wouldn't it] she wants to try again but she doesn't want another boy, you get pregnant the same time just swap, but you get what you're given. [Helen_1_2]

Psychological health appears to involve more than just efforts at maternal bonding. Women also acknowledge the personal aspect of emotional/psychological health as an integral part of the maternity experience. It is becoming an increasing aspect of the maternity experience to acknowledge that psychological health is as important as physical health. Some writers suggest that this is located in medical expert's attempts to reassert control within a landscape of increasing choice for women,[9] but it is in addition a possible consequence of living within a therapy-saturated culture where the relationship between the body and the mind is clearly acknowledged.[10] Women informed by *experts* in the form of healthcare professionals, the media and parenting magazines are increasingly aware of the impact of psychological distress on both themselves and related pregnancy outcomes. Women themselves expect to be at the mercy of their sweeping hormones, as this is how **normal pregnant women** are traditionally displayed.[4,11] Despite the apparent excess of discourse within the popular pregnancy literature,[7] Mary seems hesitant and concerned about whether her emotional feelings and responses are a normal reaction, and so firmly attributes them to an external source – hormones – early in the narrative. Women are unsure how this contemporary model of a psychological pregnancy should be depicted, they expect some hormonal/emotional reaction to the pregnancy but seem to express a concern that they are unsure at what point they become **abnormal pregnant women** and it becomes a problem.

OK a lot of sweeping hormones you get to that ten weeks and you know you dissolve into tears at things that are on the telly and I suppose that has been more but still not as I still really haven't been as sensitive as I thought I might have been you know . . . I think probably when you get to about three months you get over the more hormone swings and . . . and now I notice that I'll be fine for days and days and days and days and then I'll just get one evening and just like that I'll just . . . feel really irritable and cross and **worried** absolutely **paranoid** absolutely worried about things that may happen or the effect that it might have on me and Matt and you know irrational really . . . you know good to have a bit of a cry [I: mm] and let yourself go and it passes really but that's only every week or so. [Mary_1_3]

Jan's account also refers to fears that her emotional response to a previous pregnancy was abnormal.

> I think you change and something that used to make me very emotional, which is probably pregnancy hormones when I was expecting Ellie I didn't know the sex . . . I used to come home, come home in tears, the babies healthy and they keep saying 'I bet you want a girl, I bet you do' and Barbara came to see me my midwife and I think just fell on her crying, people keep saying 'you must want a girl and I'm not bothered Barbara' she must have thought I was mad, looking back I used to say such mad things, strange things. [Jan_1_1]

The complexity of the women's responses around their responsibilities to their babies is clear. The early narratives located the *fetus* as an active influence within the women's narratives creating the **pregnant woman**. This then appears to impose a set of rules to which they are expected to conform, including rules about the body and the emotions, in order to be a **normal pregnant woman**. The difficulty for women here is that the discourses are at times themselves confused, leaving women unsure of the emotional standard they need to attain to be a **normal pregnant woman**.

A consistent theme in these early pregnancy narratives is that women are influenced by *ideologies of mothering*, which display the identity of **a mother** through behaviours/characteristics identified as mothering functions; nurturing, advocacy, protection, responsibility for a dependant that relies almost exclusively on the biological mother, child-centred, emotionally-involving and accountable. There is a clearly defined schema (the images of identity a subject has) of motherhood with defined functions, behaviours and characteristics, which the **good mother** identity is striving to attain in relation to the *fetus*. The *GP expert's* location of some women as **abnormal pregnant women** covertly suggests that they are already failing to fulfil the most basic mothering functions of nurturing, advocacy and protection, creating tension between a **good mother** and **bad mother** identity. For others some of these functions seem more easily fulfilled. However, the **good mother** ideology, which supports notions of maternal instinct and connection/bonding, seems more difficult for all these women to attain. The **good mother** views this as a failure and a maternal inadequacy, with fears that it could in the long-term threaten the well-being of their unborn child, either physically or emotionally; consequently she locates herself as a **bad mother**.

PROMOTING MOTHERHOOD/RELEGATING FATHERHOOD

As shown, women personalise and own their pregnancies from a very early point in pregnancy. They display a responsibility to the fetus that involves making the right decisions for care and delivery, to ensure their baby's well-being during pregnancy alongside a safe and healthy outcome. The central role that women ascribe themselves is promoted further by the apparent exclusion of their partners. It is important to acknowledge the support of this exclusion by a care system that focuses on the mother and her well-being, in turn securing the babies' well-being, but as an unintended side effect excluding the father from the decision-making and responsibility sphere. This was acknowledged by Polly.

> [O]bviously for the father to see on the screen for the first time because I think it becomes a bit more real to both of you when you actually see it [I: and that's important] absolutely for him to be involved because you know all of these changes are happening to **you** and all the attention is focussed on **you** erm and you've got to remember that because its quite easy to neglect the other partner and yet he has an equal part to play in all of this the pregnancy and the labour erm but even more so with people around you they tend to . . . It's quite nice for him to be at the scan this morning so it makes it real for him. [Polly_1_1]

Although Polly's narrative suggests that the father has an equal part to play, this contradicts her earlier narrative around decisions for place of delivery. This exclusion of the father by the pregnant woman can be read as part of an embodied mothering ideology where ideals and expectations are simply part of knowledge. Women recognise the inherent difficulties for men in experiencing a reality of pregnancy but reinforce this detachment by the ownership and decision-making that they display in early pregnancy. This appears to propose that gendered parenting roles are adopted by women and assigned to their partners from a very early point in pregnancy.

We have seen women take on many of the characteristics associated with motherhood. In contrast to the characteristics of motherhood that women seem to aspire to and describe, partners, when talked about at all, are portrayed as bystanders, ascribing them the identity of *latent father*. Mary here suggests that she is already beginning to consider herself **a mother**, an identity reinforced by the narrative *latent father* role she has assigned to Matt. Mary portrays herself as taking on **a mother** identity that prepares her for life after birth in contrast to Matt who, because he is a *latent father*, she thinks is less prepared for the role to come.

> [A]nd how you'll cope with it [I: yeah and how you will cope as a couple] I don't

really have worries there but . . . I think its going to shock Matt more than he realises [laughs] I don't think he really has much idea at all. I think he has a picture in his mind of how it's going to be. [Mary_1_3]

Despite Matt's apparent concern about the *fetus*, he remains situated by Mary as not only unprepared for parenthood but unable to relate to the physical and emotional aspects associated with pregnancy, which Mary believes renders him incapable of being 'a father' in pregnancy.

[I]f I got a sharp pain and 'oh that was' you know your ligaments and things you just suddenly get a twinge or whatever straight away he would worry about it so it must be there somewhere in his mind that something could go wrong but no he wouldn't consciously sit and think about that. [Mary_1_3]

Relegating their partners to a *latent father* role is significant in that it confers and reinforces a greater level of responsibility to women for their babies and promotion of themselves as **mothers**. Analysis of Helen's narrative provides more information about this concept of the *latent father*. Her story of her previous delivery describes her husband's behaviour. The *media* plays a role here, which through its constant barrage of images and information maps out the role of the subject and creates an expectation that those roles must be accepted and fulfilled.[7] A gendered role dichotomy, fuelled by modern parenting magazines, creates an expectation for women that their partner's role is not a fathering role but one that provides support with regard to key points in the pregnancy and particularly during labour.[7]

I mean he came last time with me and he was useless basically [I: in what way] . . . and he got there, got me on the bed and the midwife said, and I was huffing and puffing and she said would you like to look, 'no no', and I said just have a look and he said 'no I don't want to' and he decided he'd have a quick peek, he'd gone on the floor out cold [I: oh no], so then they obviously had to step over him and get on with it and I was thinking if I go with him and its going to be a long one, I'd rather him stay clear, wait outside maybe . . . its just the fact I didn't want to go to hospital on my own and nobody be there [I: yeah] I mean at least I can shout him if I need to [I: yeah] but I don't think, he may want to come in but he's often said I hope I'm 500 miles away when you go into labour which is nice isn't it?. . . but at least 5 minutes afterwards he thought it was all wonderful and glorious you know. [Helen_1_2]

Helen's narrative demonstrates that she perceives her partner's role to be one of support, and her dissatisfaction with his lack of support is apparent. These maternal narratives suggest that women are influenced by the discourses that afford partners a role to play in pregnancy but clearly not as 'fathers', which directly contrasts with the maternal discourses that shape women's roles in pregnancy.

PERFECT BABIES AND SCREENING CHOICE

The 'choice in maternity care' debate requires consideration of some of the other choices faced by women (and their partners), for example, with regard to genetic screening. It would seem a reasonable assumption that women desiring and choosing a more 'natural birth experience' might also make non-interventionalist choices with regard to screening. Further analysis of whether this was the case and how screening decisions were made seemed to offer potential in illuminating the choice concept. Women's choices, as already illustrated, are complex bound up in their previous maternity experiences (*personal knowing*), their acceptance of the authority of *the medical discourses* and *ideologies of mothering*. The role played by the *scan* in reaffirming women's **pregnant woman, normal pregnant woman** and **good mother** status has already been illustrated. This conflicts with the purpose of the *scan*, as viewed by *experts*, who consider even the early *scan* an opportunity to look for soft markers of abnormality and part of the screening process, that situates woman as **abnormal pregnant women**. Women are willingly complicit with the scan because of its role in reaffirming their identities, as Polly demonstrates below.

> I did express my concern that I obviously didn't feel pregnant and erm one way of putting my mind at ease was the fact that she gave me the scan erm and she said to me it wasn't an official scan but she could see that I was quite anxious that I didn't think I was pregnant so she would do that just to show me that there was a heart beat etc. there and that was really [important]. [Polly_1_1]

The aim of genetic screening is to allow couples to make informed reproductive choices. However, when explored through the narratives of these women, *prenatal testing* emerges as an influence that reinforces the idea that it is both natural and right to want a *perfect baby*.[12] Mary and Helen both identify the 20-week anomaly *scan* as an intervention to confirm normality: it is not given the same screening status attributed to other screening tests. Their narratives illustrate that other screening test choices are far more multifaceted than those displayed with regard to scanning. Screening underplays the emotional and experiential aspects of pregnancy that are inherent in these women's pregnancy stories. The *ideology of mothering* positions women as caring, nurturing and protective, yet screening demands a willingness to abort a damaged child. Mary feels in some way that she has to justify her decision to go for screening. *Personal knowing* plays a significant role in informing her decision, with recognition that a high-risk result would have undermined all her embodied feelings about her pregnancy, her baby and made her question the new identities that pregnancy has created. Mary's narrative depicts *a disabled child* as one that is always a baby and never fulfils its potential. It never achieves the markers of success, e.g. going to college, by which parents are judged to have been successful in their roles. For Mary a disabled child reflects a **bad mother** on two levels, the first in her failure to protect and nurture in the womb, the second, lack of achievement by which to measure her parenting success. **Abnormal motherhood** is a role given by the child that never ends; a dark journey with no light at the end. Women who bring up disabled children, however, are often perceived as highly self-sacrificing,[8] a characteristic usually associated with **good mothering**. Women are expected to be able to judge the right course of action. The conflict entrenched in Mary's narrative between the **good mother** and **bad mother** identities is exemplified in her hesitancy about what her decisions would be in the face of a negative screening outcome

> [E]ven just like having the triple test was a huge thing just for us to talk through and go through [I: and did you have it in the end] yeah yeah I did I did I still don't know if it came back it was 1 in 12,000 or something I still don't know what I would have done if you know if the ratio had been really low but I'm glad I had it. [I: What made you think what made you make the decision to have it?] Loads of things, lots of different practical issues around having a child who was severely disabled except you wouldn't know it may be a healthy little Down's child who goes to college and all sorts you don't know that's the difficulty the other thing is my cousin has got severe Down's syndrome and he's my age and he can't do anything, he's still in nappies and everything and I know what a massive impact he had on the family and they've really been through some dark times so you know it would mean a massive massive change a massive impact . . . so I thought I'd be better equipped at knowing what to do if I had some facts . . . having the facts and then making a decision based on them. [I: hard though isn't it?] Yeah because you do have to think through these things like what will I do if . . . then we go down and have a amniocentesis and then what would we do then cos the very fact you're having a test shows that you need to know for some reason. [Mary_1_3]

Helen's narrative, below, as with choices for care, demonstrates less autonomy in the choice process. Screening is a professional discourse that many *experts* feel compelled to advocate for women's own and societal good.[5] Helen seems to neither want nor feel able to challenge that. The decision to maintain a pregnancy for Helen is based on her judgements about what constitutes *a disabled child* and on her ability to cope and be a **good mother**.

> They do all these tests, the doctors do them regardless, I mean you have your options of having them done or you don't, I think if they're offering them then you take them I mean the earlier you know there's anything the matter then the better really [I: yeah so it wasn't a difficult decision] oh no they said at the booking in clinic do you want this that or the other and I said 'oh yeah I'll have them all' as I said the earlier I know there's something the matter the better. [I: How would that affect your feelings about your pregnancy?] It obviously didn't really . . . if it was disabled, it would depend as to what sort of severity, if I went if I went to my 20-week scan and they said its got a foot missing or a hand missing or whatever that wouldn't bother me, I don't think it would bother me [coughs] but if they said it was something more serious then maybe I don't know spina bifida or whatever then . . . I'd have to think twice . . . its a full time job isn't it [I: mm mm] I mean my personal point of view I don't think I could do that. [Helen_1_2]

Polly makes a decision not to have screening based on the perceived precious-ness of her pregnancy and her need to be a mother. The risk of not getting pregnant again outweighs the concerns about disability. This decision is not made lightly, clearly creates anxiety and demonstrates the same conflict between **good mother** and **bad mother** articulated by Mary.

> [A]t this moment in time the biggest concern for me is the screening for Down's syndrome because on seeing the consultant she was very adamant that I took the screening and also the test and when I asked the question why all she could really say was that it was predominantly to do with my age and that there is a high-risk factor at my age of 36 erm . . . and that she would recommend every woman of my age to go through this screening process. So that's the biggest worry and concern to me at this moment because I'm quite adamant that I don't want to go through it. [I: So what makes you so adamant, what makes you think you don't want that screening?] Because they couldn't give me a hundred percent erm . . . on either the screening or the other test erm . . . to actually yes you are carrying a Down's Syndrome baby erm and if they could give me a hundred percent accuracy then I may be swayed toward it but its also the fact

> that I also know there's a risk involved with the second test of actually going through miscarriage and erm obviously getting to my age now and trying for a baby, miscarriage is the last thing I want to go through so its quite an important factor for me not to put the baby at risk. [Polly _1_1]

Polly is able to resist the *expert* who clearly advocates that the correct choice would be to accept screening; however, Helen's unquestioning acceptance of the dominant discourse around screening is reinforced by Jan.

> I've gone through some screening, I'm getting a blood test back on Monday . . . its more like worrying about Down's cos my friend . . . her first baby was Down's and she was younger than me a few years younger we were all a bit shocked about that . . . .its a bit close to home its frightened me a bit . . . paranoid person [laughs]. [Jan_1_1]

What is apparent in these narratives, contrary to previous literature,[13] is that women are capable of ranking their needs with regard to screening choices. With regard to choice, decisions are based on individual circumstances and subjective perceptions of *a disabled child*. The influence of the *fetus* and the need to be a **good mother**, which is more difficult in the face of disability as for Helen 'if they said it was something more serious then maybe I don't know spina bifida or whatever then . . . I'd have to think twice . . . its a full-time job isn't it', consistently infuses these narratives.

EXPERTS AND EXPERTISE

The well-documented sociological history of childbirth recognises changes over time in the continuing conflict between women, doctors and midwives about who knows best and an exercise in power.[5] Current policy claims to return power to women, proffering a model of maternity care that is women-centred, premised on the view that women make informed and considered choices. The very foundation of this research, demonstrates that structural changes have occurred in the delivery of maternity services; perhaps more fundamental, however, is whether a transformation in the power relations between these groups is really taking place. The integral influential role played by the *GP expert/gatekeeper* in influencing and controlling woman's maternity choices, as well as *personal knowing*, acceptance of the *medical discourse* and the need to be a **good mother** have already been highlighted. What is apparent from these interview narratives is that *expert* intervention remains largely undisputed. More interesting perhaps is how women define who maternity experts are and how those definitions impact on their decision-making. Several experts are defined within these early narratives; the narratives about ultrasound scanning locate the *scan* as an expert, providing reassurance of normality and a healthy pregnancy. As may be expected, however, the main reference to maternity expertise refers to midwives and obstetricians who are obvious individual *expert* characters within the narratives, and women's deference to the *experts*, as in Polly's account below, to assure the well-being of their pregnancies locates women as **maternity patients**.

> I think my outlook on it is if the doctor and midwife are happy with the progress of my pregnancy then I'm quite happy. [Polly_1_1]

Midwives and doctors are at other times conceptualised differently. Mary has made a choice to have midwifery-led care but to deliver at the acute hospital unit. Mary's narrative only situates herself as a potential **maternity patient** requiring *expert* advice in the face of a serious event. The *expert* that has the ability to reassure her **normal pregnant woman** status is the midwife, but she also has the capacity to locate her as a **maternity patient** by referring her to the doctor.

> [I: So if anything happened if something happened that you were unsure about . . . what would be your first point of contact?] Erm . . . I don't know really, depending on what it was I may well check with friends and family if I thought I suppose really it could be anything serious I suppose I'd ring the midwife, ring the Health Centre and ask them [I: mm mm] for advice. [Mary_1_3]

Sally echoes Mary's sentiments about the midwife.

> I'd probably contact the midwife I think or the doctor but probably the midwife because they're doing it all the time . . . the doctors dealing with so many different things and I'd rather just go to someone who deals with that one specific thing and speak to them about it . . . because that's all they do day in day out and you can tell by the er . . . they got a lot of experience and they know what's what . . . but I'd just . . . think I'll just go to my midwife, a bit like if I had a problem with my eyes I'd go to my optician not my doctor. [Sally _1_1]

Helen's narrative response to the same question, however, suggests differently. She views the midwife and the doctor as interdependent and working together, rather than dichotomous as suggested by the other women's stories. In some ways once again the GP acts as the *gatekeeper* to the appropriate maternity services. This seems to be in opposition to Helen's choice of a birth-centre delivery, at which care is provided wholly by midwives. A possible explanation for this is that Helen, as we have seen previously, considers herself a **normal pregnant woman** and consequently she does not need medical input. Identification of a problem, however, would locate her as a potentially **abnormal pregnant woman** and necessitate the need for a *medical expert* to identify her as a **maternity patient**.

> The doctor. [I: so you would choose to see the doctor, you could phone the midwife directly but you would choose the doctor?] Yeah of course, you can talk to them and see what your options are or . . . what to do next or whatever. [I: Why would it be the doctor? Not that there is anything wrong with that] No particular reason just because they're round the corner, they sort of do doctors, midwives together, they work together don't they? [Helen_1_2]

Polly awards both the doctor and the midwife *expert* status, situating them both as *experts* who can confirm her **normal pregnant woman** identity but later distinguishes the midwife as the pregnancy *'expert'* and the one she would contact with her initial concerns.

> Yeah yeah, because I feel that they're the experts (doctors and midwives) in that that's what they specialise in and they see this every single day, this for me is something completely new and so if they said to me if I have anything and I see them every 4 weeks and they turn round and say its quite normal don't worry about it you know all women go through this then I will be quite happy that will put my mind at rest . . . [I: Do you think it would make any difference whether it was a doctor or a midwife?] Erm . . . yes I think it would and I think it would probably get down to the midwife because as I say that's what she specialises in every day of her working career so you know she comes across so many different issues and so many different women with different experiences. [Polly_1_1]

Polly's narrative supports Helen's, that the midwife is the practitioner to go to as **normal pregnant woman**, and thus locates the midwife, as she has been traditionally portrayed, as the healthcare professional most able to confirm and reassure normality. This fits with the depiction of midwives as 'guardians of the normal'[14] and a midwifery model of care, which emphasises the naturalness and normality of pregnancy and birth. This narrative, however, still fails to support a model of care where the woman has control and power, relying on the expertise of her own body. Bryar's claim that women shift their thinking about childbirth according to different contexts and circumstances[15] is supported by

Mary's comments about her choices for place of delivery. Despite feeling happy to be cared for by midwives and reassured by the normality of her pregnancy, Mary's choice for place of delivery continues to be infused by *medical discourse* and the claim that a hospital with medical presence remains the safest place to give birth, despite a recognition through policy that this claim cannot be justified and a plethora of available literature supporting that view.

> Yessss . . . erm I suppose I mean as times going on it's erm I sort of wonder you see I know the birth-centre they don't it's just midwifery led [I: yes] and as time's going on I feel more confident that that would have been alright but with it everything being such a first for me you know. [Mary_1_3]

Polly's narrative further highlights the role of *experts*. Despite women's acknowledgement that the midwife has the power to locate them as maternity patients, the *midwife expert* is firmly linked with the identity of **normal pregnant woman**, and the *medical expert* with the identity of **abnormal pregnant woman**.

> Something that's wrong, rather than a midwife is oh yeah general yes and everyday thing you get pregnant you see a midwife you just put the two together it's a natural you see a consultant you automatically think is there something wrong. [Polly_1_1]

Mary here suggests that *expert* knowledge is also provided from other sources including *personal knowing, official pregnancy literature* and *magazines*, as well as *friends and family*, as in Mary's narrative.

> Erm . . . I've got younger sisters, my youngest sister is 12 so I've always been around babies quite a lot but a lot of my friends my age have just gone through all this so they're the ones, so hearing what they say . . . not really my Mum cos she's not in your face with things like that and she knows that things have changed a lot and you do get some people telling you saying certain things to you but you don't let them bother you, and books I've read loads of books. [Mary_1_3]

Sally also refers to *books* and *magazines* as well as *friends* as *experts*.

> I bought a book, Miriam Stoppard book, which seems is really good and I've also found useful the information that I get from my doctors and my midwife when I go you know the information things and I read some bits of it and stuff like that they've been brilliant really I've got enough information really the

> bounty book I've got a lot of the information I'm getting from there . . . so yeah you get information from doctors, midwives and from friends. [Sally_1_1]

It seems that whilst women enjoy reading these magazines they do not replace the expertise provided by midwives and doctors. *Personal knowing* is not considered as informative or reliable as *expert knowing*.

> Er . . . I've got **the book,** I got given the book and that goes week by week, tells you what you should be doing and where you should be going for this that and the other and you know . . . but as I say I've had two already sort of I know those things, it has slightly changed since I had my last one you know . . . [I: So where would say most of your information about your pregnancy comes from?] The majority of it comes from having the other two and as I said the little book that I got given and magazines, I get quite a few of the mother and baby magazines, I quite like reading some of the stories in there. [Did they give you a lot of information at the booking clinic?]Not a great deal no, not a great deal, I think with me having previous pregnancies its just a case of tick the boxes as you go along [I: mm] . . . I mean I had to ask quite a few questions and she was kind of looking at me as if to say you should know that and I didn't. [Helen_1_2]

Throughout women's narratives expertise is consistent. *Experts*, however, take many different forms and are accessed depending on a woman's personal assessment of the situation. Different experts, such as midwives and doctors, are often combined within the women's stories to signify expertise and are segregated dependant on individual events. This could suggest that choice can only ever be an evolving decision and that choice of lead carer/expert cannot be the singular decision that it is presented as in early pregnancy.

SUMMARY

The narratives identified in early pregnancy demonstrate how the confirmation of a pregnancy causes women to adopt a new **pregnant woman** identity. This status locates the *fetus* as a powerful influence and initiates the transition to motherhood. This invests women with a personal responsibility to act appropriately in pregnancy, make responsible choices to maintain the pregnancy and ensure their baby's well-being. Tensions for women exist as they are situated by the various discourses and influences that surround them in pregnancy as **responsible/irresponsible, normal/abnormal pregnant women,** and as they aspire to promote themselves as **good mothers.** Whilst the narratives around screening demonstrate that women are capable of ranking their desires and concerns to make choices, that choice continues to only exist within the frameworks defined by *experts, culturally mediated discourses, ideologies and standards*. Whilst some of these influences offer the promise of choice, others clearly restrain it, presenting choice in maternity care as a complex phenomenon, that is not merely based on the type of pregnancy and birth experience desired.

REFERENCES

1 Chou F, Lin L, Cooney A. Psychosocial factors relating to nausea, vomiting, and fatigue in early pregnancy. *J Nurs Scholarship.* 2003; **35**(2): 119–25.

2 Munch S. Chicken or the egg? The biological psychological controversy surrounding hyperemesis gravidarum. *Soc Sci Med.* 2002; **55**(7): 1267–78.

3 Gatrell C. *Hard Labour: the sociology of parenthood.* Maidenhead: Open University Press; 2005.

4 Gross H. Pregnancy: a healthy state. In: Ussher JM, editor. *Women's Health: contemporary international health perspectives.* Leicester: The British Psychological Society; 2000.

5 Kent J. *Social Perspectives on Pregnancy and Childbirth for Midwives, Nurses and the Caring Professions.* Buckingham: Open University Press; 2000.

6 Oakley A. *From Here to Maternity: becoming a mother.* Harmondsworth: Penguin; 1981.

7 Sunderland J. *Gendered Discourses.* Basingstoke: Palgrave Macmillan; 2004.

8 Singh I. Doing their jobs: mothering with Ritalin in a culture of mother-blame. *Soc Sci Med.* 2004; **59**(6): 1193–205.

9 Weaver J. Childbirth. In: Ussher JM, editor. *Women's Health: contemporary international health perspectives.* Leicester: The British Psychological Society; 2000.

10 Steward W. A 'therapy culture' may be doing more harm than good. *Nursing Times.* 2004; **100**(18): 16.

11 Crawford M, Unger R. *Women and Gender.* 4th ed. New York: McGraw Hill; 2004.

12 Chadwick R. The perfect baby. In: Chadwick R, editor. *Ethics, Reproduction and Genetic Control.* London: Routledge; 1990.

13 Shickle D, Chadwick R. The ethics of screening: is screeningitis an incurable disease? *J Med Ethics.* 1994; **20**(1): 12–18.

14 Downe S. Who defines abnormality? *Nursing Times.* 1991; **87**(18): 22.

15 Bryar R. *Theory for Midwifery Practice.* Basingstoke: Macmillan; 1995.

CHAPTER 6

'The labour of pregnancy': late pregnancy and impending labour

32–36 WEEKS

The following section presents the narrative themes identified in late pregnancy. Many of the themes identified here build on the themes identified in early pregnancy. As pregnancy progresses many of the identities and influences surrounding women during pregnancy are reinforced. Narratives, as would be expected, are gestation specific and so the themes emerge from a slightly different context. Themes consistent with early pregnancy include:

➤ the new identity: pregnant back to non-pregnant
➤ identity, ownership and choice
➤ promoting motherhood/relegating fatherhood.

A new theme is identified specific to impending labour:
➤ labour expectations.

Other themes less relevant to this stage of pregnancy have disappeared including:
➤ the GP gatekeeper
➤ physical pregnancy
➤ perfect babies and screening choice.

Experts and expertise and the new identity, naturalness, responsibility and emotions, rather than being individual themes now infuse the other identified themes.

The new identity: from pregnant back to non-pregnant

The role of the *fetus* in reinforcing the **pregnant woman** identity continues to be consistent in the narratives. There is an evident change in their physical appearance as the fetus referred to by Jane.

> I'm very obviously pregnant. [Jane_2_1]

This changing shape also facilitates recognition and acknowledgement from others of their **pregnant woman** status.

> Completely different because you can see that I'm pregnant and I feel so proud when I'm walking around . . . and people stop you and it's the attention you get and it's lovely . . . and they want to talk about you and the baby and you come out glowing with this sense of pride. [Polly_2_1]

The fear of returning to **non-pregnant woman** is diminished, although Helen's account shows a readiness to return to **non-pregnant woman** created by the birth of the baby.

> I am [ready to deliver], I've had my bags packed since 26 weeks. I got my last bits yesterday and I'm just waiting now. [Helen_2_2]

Sophie expresses a similar readiness to return to **non-pregnant woman**. Both of these narratives suggest that women need to feel prepared for birth and they intimate that physical preparation facilitates psychological preparation.

> All the clothes are prepared now and the baby's bedroom's done I've got my bottles and everything so I'm ready. [Sophie_2_1]

Mary's account embodies the suggestion that physical and psychological preparations for birth are intimately connected. The mothering role following birth seems acknowledged as something different to the current **mother** role she is engaged in. A feasible interpretation is that the mothering role that women aspire and create for themselves in pregnancy is different, particularly in emotional content, to the mothering that women feel they will have to fulfil following birth.

> Only in that it suddenly it made everything ever so kind of real in a sense of . . . you see the other thing when they admitted me, I was getting regular tightenings like every 10 minutes for about 24 hours or something and they were sort of

muttering about that all the time and all night long I had visions of going into labour and I suddenly thought crikey, you know and they did say it may be at this stage it sort of comes early and this kind of thing and that sort of shocks you [I: yeah] in that oh, I've nothing ready, I'm not prepared for this emotionally, I'm still in my head, I've still got all this way to go . . . I've been sort of getting a few bits and bobs ready just in case. [Mary_2_2]

Polly, enjoying being a **pregnant woman**, is reluctant to relinquish that status.

Erm, now its feels exactly the same as probably when I was 14 weeks. I still feel really well I'm still enjoying being pregnant. [Polly_2_1]

Helen's story continues as she goes on to suggest that the *fetus* will be active in contradicting her desire to return to her **non-pregnant woman** identity.

I think it will be late, I've just got a feeling it will be late, I do. I do, I think it's going to be awkward and really late. You know it'll only come when it's ready. I did think it would come early but . . . [Helen_2_2]

This short narrative above is quite complex, Helen is anxious to end the pregnancy but this conflicts with her desire expressed in early pregnancy to deliver at the birth centre. This choice can only be facilitated by the baby arriving at a later gestation than her previous pregnancies. This supports the earlier suggestion that choice is a complex phenomenon that evolves throughout the pregnancy, with gestation-specific events and experience, dictating women's feelings and decisions as pregnancy progresses. Helen's ongoing *physical symptoms* in pregnancy inform her desire to return to a **non-pregnant woman**, perhaps due to a need for reassurance that the baby is normal and well despite her ill health, and thus confirming Helen as a **good mother**. This appears to supersede her desire for a birth-centre delivery.

[N]ot been feeling too well . . . I've been like all the way through, lots of problems, low blood pressure, headache, heartburn, you name it I've had it. I'm hating it, it's been the worst one of all three of them. The other two weren't too bad this one's just . . . so horrible, definitely no more, definitely. I couldn't cope with another 9 months of feeling like this . . . I've had headaches all the way through the whole thing and they say it's caused by my low blood pressure and I just have to slow down. It's a bit difficult when you've got two kids and you don't get any time to yourself. [Helen_2_2]

Helen's account locates the *fetus* as the cause of the physical problems and suggests that the *fetus* has a part to play in dictating its arrival. This clearly merits further interpretation. The *fetus*, which in early pregnancy created a **pregnant woman** identity, is now ascribed a role in Helen's return to **non-pregnant woman**. Helen's labelling of the *fetus* not only ascribes the *fetus* agency and self will, it also attributes it with characteristics. A later gestation will actually facilitate Helen's choice for delivery, yet Helen still labels the *fetus* as awkward, building a multifaceted picture of negative feelings. This narrative portrays the *fetus* as having rational, decision-making capabilities, when it is still a dependant being with no existence beyond the mother. No conclusive scientific evidence identifies the fetus as the catalyst to the onset of labour, but Helen ascribes her *fetus* a defined and active role to play in terms of pregnancy events and outcomes. It seems that this baby will be conceptualised as awkward whenever Helen delivers. Awkward because it is maintaining Helen's pregnancy when she would rather deliver or awkward because it prevents her from delivering early. This baby creates tensions for Helen because she is trying to be a **good mother** to both her existing children and this baby. *Experts*, through medical knowledge and the *physical symptoms of her pregnancy*, have situated her as an **abnormal pregnant woman**, advising her to act in a certain way to ensure her well-being and so her baby's. Adhering to their advice forces her to be a **bad mother** to her other children. Attributing her *fetus* with an active role allows Helen to devolve some of the responsibility for the perceived failures of a **bad mother**.

IDENTITY, OWNERSHIP AND CHOICE

The intricacy of Helen's pregnancy experience is augmented by the role of the *experts* in labelling her as an **abnormal pregnant woman**. She feels that this unfairly represents her as a **bad mother**, despite her having always delivered healthy babies (**good mother**). Although she has been given choice, it is restricted; she feels as a consequence unfairly categorised and as a result controlled. The health professionals are lumped into one category and referred to as 'they', although in this case she is primarily talking about the doctor as a *medical expert* controlling her choices, and he is depicted as bad. Helen defines herself as a **normal pregnant woman** constructed though *personal knowing*, and feels cheated that she is unable to have a true choice. Whilst her experiential knowledge reassures her that there will not be any problems at delivery, she permits *expert medical knowing*, which plays on fears about the safety of her baby, to dominate, diminishing her personal ownership of the pregnancy. Helen reinforces her early pregnancy concerns that her choices are actually to ensure *expert* attendance at delivery.

> I haven't had any problems with my other pregnancies so I couldn't see why I couldn't go there, but like I tried to explain to the doctor, a woman who's 40-weeks pregnant can have complications, so a woman who's 35-weeks pregnant can be straight forward, but they don't look at it like that. [I: I suppose what they're thinking of is the special care unit] Well that's what he says, no because there's no doctors up there. [I: So then if you had the choice, and I said the choice is at 37 weeks you'll have to go to Hull or 38 weeks you can go to the birth centre] I'd go to the birth centre, yeah I would yeah [I: Much as you've felt awful] Yeah I would I'd rather go there, I've heard the other one's real nice but I'd still rather go there it's nearer, more convenient. This is it I'm thinking am I going to get there in time. [Helen_2_2]

Helen has already placed a responsibility on the *fetus* for her delivery. Claims that her propensity to premature delivery is hereditary further devolve the responsibility. It's not that she's a failure, an **abnormal pregnant woman** or a **bad mother** it is just something that she is powerless to prevent.

> It runs in the family, I was 7 weeks early, my middle sister was 5 weeks early, my eldest sister was 6 weeks early. My sisters have had kids and they've both been 2/3 weeks early . . . I think it just runs in the family. [I: So it's not been specific reasons?] No, no, I think my mum had me at 33 weeks and she had high blood pressure with me . . . but the other two just came when they were ready to come I think. [Helen_2_2]

Mary's account tells a different story, but equally demonstrates choice to be a privilege that can be rescinded. She has developed *physical symptoms of pregnancy*, which necessitate surveillance and potential intervention, and hence play a role in situating Mary as an **abnormal pregnant woman**. Mary's experience justifies her early pregnancy choice to deliver at the acute unit in case of problems. The midwife as an *expert* has defined Mary as a **maternity patient**. Problems have arisen in her pregnancy and choosing antenatal midwifery-led care has not detracted from her or her baby's well-being. Therefore, she made the responsible decisions of a **good mother**.

> I did want to have midwifery-led care . . . they've all been the same midwives which is really nice, I think that makes a big difference . . . [I: Have you felt confident in seeing the midwives, you've not felt at any point, oh I wish I'd seen the GP?] No, no I feel every confidence, and as I say the second anything is sort of out of line she was straight onto it, checking blood pressure and we'll do this, walked in and she said oh hi Mary, how are you doing, she said the first

girl at 9.00 has just fainted on me, the second girl I've just had to admit . . . she said you're going to be straightforward, and I said I hope so and I wasn't but she's still so, you know, she wasn't oh now I've got to go and do this and you know and she was oh never mind I've got to do this and that, really smashing. [Mary_2_2]

Other women reassert their rationale for the choices made in early pregnancy based on their individualised perceptions of risk generated by the continued infusion of the *medical discourse*, i.e. making choices to ensure the well-being of their babies and promote their **good mother** identities. Kate, despite preferring the birth-centre, chooses the acute unit.

Yeah, well I do want the birth centre but if anything goes wrong then I don't want any doubt about it. [Kate_2_1]

Sally equally reinforces her original choice.

I'm quite happy to come here (acute unit) I think there's a lot of people who know what they are doing and no I'm quite happy and it makes sense . . . erm I think if there was anything wrong everything's handy doctor and all that sort of stuff, whatever you need is all nearby . . . I know I haven't had any problems with my pregnancy but I just rather be in this environment for my first time. [Sally_2_1]

Jane is able to justify her choice through the experience of her sister-in-law. Her account remains less influenced by *medical discourse*, and quality of care is an important consideration judged, however, by the input perceived necessary to facilitate **good mother** skills following delivery.

I think that suite (birth centre) through there is absolutely lovely and . . . my sister-in-law, she had hers at the R . . . and even though it was at the new place she said it was absolutely awful . . . [I: Why do you think that was?] I just think it's because they've been so busy and she was in a side room and she wanted help with breast feeding and it was like, she'd been breast feeding for most of the afternoon, nobody had been to see her, and she just wanted to go home and nobody had been to see her and nobody was helping her, and I think coming down to it they were just so busy but that didn't help her. [I: So that's reinforced your decision for the Birth Centre?] Yeah, absolutely . . . I've got absolutely no qualms about making that decision. [Jane_2_1]

The **good mother/bad mother** dichotomy is exhibited throughout and across all the women's narratives. Mary, now labelled as an **abnormal pregnant woman**, needs to reassert her **good mother** identity through narrative claims that she was well until 30-weeks pregnant, describing the 'wobbly moment' when she fears she is losing a grasp of that identity. Mary's narrative, unlike Helen's, apportions no blame to the fetus. Mary rather questions her innate sense of her own body (*personal knowing*). Her narrative implies denial that there was a problem, evident in the alternative explanations she offers for her raised blood pressure. An inherent contradiction of identities exists for Mary here. Failed *personal knowing* locates Mary as a **bad mother** failing to be an advocate for the baby's well-being, an identity reinforced by the handover of the nurturing and protecting role inherent in good mothering to the *experts*. Mary no longer has a choice in decisions; her care is now dictated by the fact that she is now a **maternity patient**, which necessitates surrendering of choice and control. Her unquestioning acceptance of this handover of choice and control, however, reasserts her **good mother** identity.

> Erm, it was moving along quite nicely really, up to about say 30 weeks when I had blood pressure problems . . . I mean looking back I think I can tell now when it's sort of going up, the difficulty is with you not being pregnant before you don't know what's what, you know and like every night after tea I'd be getting this pounding in my head but I just thought you get extra blood volume don't you [I: yeah yeah] at the end of the day and things but no I didn't feel unwell, there was no indication really. [I: So was it just a general antenatal check then you went to?] Yeah, yeah, I checked it at work a couple of times during the week and I thought oh that's a bit up but you sort of think well I'm at work I've just done a shift and its gonna be up a little bit and then I went . . . she said we'll just get you into the Antenatal Day Unit at Castle Hill and it was about the same there and then it was 160/100 over the weekend so . . . Yeah which was erh, that was really the only sort of wobbly moment really because as you're sat there I was looking at the dial and I saw it start to go to the 160 mark and I thought 'oh no' its really gone up . . . I've suddenly developed this problem because my blood pressure was 100/60 every week and she said its suddenly gone up this much she said erm we'll need to watch you closely because I've got a feeling you're on the brink of maybe pre-eclampsia. [Mary_2_2]

Like Helen, Mary abdicates some responsibility for her **abnormal pregnant woman/bad mother** status by attributing the problem to a hereditary condition.

[M]y mum had it with me I don't know if it's familial but erm she said we'll just monitor you closely. [Mary_2_2]

Mary continues to assert her **good mother** role, suggesting she has done enough to protect and nurture her baby to ensure its survival, even if premature. Interestingly, the *expert* of choice here is the *pregnancy book*, rather than the health professionals who indirectly elevate her **bad mother** identity.

I thought I was at 30 weeks, I thought everything would probably be okay and I think that week I'd read in my book that if the baby was born now it would stand an excellent chance of survival and this kind of thing. [Mary_2_2]

Early pregnancy demonstrated how women individually make choices based on a plethora of orbiting social and cultural discourses, as well as being influenced by the *fetus*, the *GP gatekeeper*, expertise in many different forms and experiential knowledge. As pregnancy progresses this choice is reinforced and justified by several women. For others who become **maternity patients,** however, it becomes an illusory concept removed or dictated by pregnancy-specific events.

LABOUR EXPECTATIONS

Thoughts and worries about labour, which are not really expressed in early pregnancy, now begin to become more prominent. Mary narrates her thoughts about labour and her perception that it will be out of her control. Coping and control appear intimately related and women articulate them as both physical and emotional events. Her perception of labour is based on influential *experienced labourer* discourses that surround her, these are predominantly 'horror stories'.

I think it was just that I thought it was way away, I knew it was coming, I'd read lots about it, psychologically you think you're prepared but I mean you're bound to be frightened to some extent because it's something that is happening out of your control that's never happened to you before . . . it's just a bit scary really [laugh] how you're gonna cope, if you'll cope, what'll happen, you know all the different things you always hear about all the horror stories . . . my auntie and then my dad's wife she had two bad births as well and I think when people do go onto you about it a bit and how horrendous it is, you know it does sort of . . . I mean it must be so difficult to explain what it is like but there's no other way of understanding it is there. [Mary_2_2]

The *experienced labourer* accounts, which inform Mary's account above, juxtapose with her desire to have the normal, fulfilling emotional experience that some women describe and is portrayed in some of the *media and pregnancy literature*.[1] Negative *experienced labourer* discourses generate similar expectations of labour as necessitating intervention and it seems feasible that Mary's expectations of lack of control are generated with these stories. Mary's fear of labour, her perception that pregnancy and birth are inherently risky and her construction of labour as a natural but unpredictable and undisciplined experience illuminate her choice for delivery site. Delivery at an acute unit does not inherently imply a willingness to relinquish all control but rather a desire for control over when to relinquish control. Mary expects a point in her labour where she is no longer able to act as an advocate or be responsible for the well-being of herself (**uncontrolled labourer**) and consequently her baby and her choice implies a willingness to hand over control at that point, promoting herself as a **good mother**.

> I imagine a lot of pain but hope that I can cope with it, the only thing I don't want it to turn into an experience where it becomes a really big trauma for me you know what I mean . . . you want it to be a positive experience as well don't you [I – yeah absolutely] and people, there are lots of people that do tell you that as well and course it's really painful but at the same time it's an amazing experience to go through so yes I'm expecting lots of pain, I'm not expecting it to be easy . . . I'm expecting things to happen that I don't expect to happen, erm . . . but I want it to sort of stay within that realm of almost . . . this is all normal, it's what's supposed to happen, it's physically wildly out of my control, you know this experience but I get something good out of it as well . . . if they told me I needed a caesarean section then I would be really disappointed. [Mary_2_2]

Jane's narrative emphasises the constructed nature of her first experience of labour and fears of how she will react, underpinned by similar discourses to Mary.

> I don't know really, I think I've heard too many people and their stories that I think that's part of my trouble really, that I don't really know what to expect. I've been reading about the signs and things like that erm . . . but if I'm honest I don't really know actually. I'm just going to have to see how it goes and I know it's going to be painful and things like that erm . . . I'm just going to have to wait and see. [Jane_2_1]

For Helen her choices for delivery are bound up with a slightly different concept of control. Attempts to maintain control in labour are based on her own *experienced labourer* discourse where her previous deliveries have not created feelings of control. *Cultural norms* suggest that society feels uncomfortable witnessing the expression of basic human emotions and this paints a picture of women out of control in labour as something unattractive/animalistic.[2] Hence women feel that being out of control is an unacceptable way to behave in labour and are pressured to conform to the serene Madonna-esque picture of a **good mother** even in labour.

> Very quick ones, the second one was awful, we only just got there 8.30 to hospital, she was born at 8.35 and it was just a case of on the bed and out she popped. From that perspective it was rather quick and a bit of a shock to the system, I expected to be there for hours and hours, no out she popped and that was it . . . I think it's from a past experience really, I would sort of say I expect the same sort of labour as I had with the other two. [Helen_2_2]

Some women's accounts reveal that choices are made based on the availability of *epidurals*, which play a potentially important role in facilitating the **controlled labourer**.

> I'm going to the main unit it's just if I want an epidural which I had last time you see [I: right] I want to have that option. [Sophie_2_1]

Though there is an expectation that labour will be painful and recognition that some expression of pain is acceptable it still is expected to be within a frame of control, e.g. quiet moaning is acceptable but loud screaming and swearing is not. Midwives have traditionally encouraged women to control pushing in the second stage of labour to facilitate a smooth, less traumatic, delivery both for baby and mother. Hence both *cultural and expert discourses* bolster notions of a **controlled labourer**. Sally, like Mary, supports a willing hand-over of decision-making and elements of control to the *expert*.

> I'm not sure what my pain threshold going to be like and whether I'll need an epidural but from what they've said the midwife will guide me. [Sally_2_1]

Helen's narrative illustrates other labour concerns that impact on choice. These suggest that despite her claims to normality, Helen clearly worries about abnormal events in labour, possibly manifested by her categorisation from early pregnancy as an **abnormal pregnant woman**, which inherently denies her personal control. Her choices for the birth centre as the nearest site assured of *expert* input have already been discussed. Her earlier narrative also suggests that a quicker admission may also facilitate a greater level of control. Her choice may equally be based on hopes for a less interventionist approach to her delivery and affirmation of her **normal pregnant woman** identity. Helen once again utilises the narrative to promote her **good mother** identity displaying characteristics of protection and self-sacrifice.

> My worst fear is caesarean section, I don't know why but uh . . . it frightens me I don't know why, why . . . I've just never wanted a section, no. I think that would be my worse fear if they said you're gonna have a section I'd think oh no. I don't know really it's just the thought of being cut open . . . it's just the thought of having it. I'm just not keen on it. Its difficult cos even if you don't want one at the end of the day it's about your baby isn't it? If I had to have, if they said to me, well I'm going to have to cut you open or there's a chance it could go wrong then cut me open, I wouldn't sort of say, I'm not going to let you do it I'd say go ahead and do it. [Helen_2_2]

Kate mirrors this self-sacrificing role of a **good mother**. Her narrative suggests a complete absence of control – 'If it needs to be done it needs to be done you can't stop it'.

> No I'm alright about it (labour) at the moment, my only worry is when I come out will I be able to manage living on my own . . . as long as I don't have a caesarean section I'm sure we'll be able to manage . . . [I: Would it bother you if you had to have a section?] No not particularly . . . If it needs to be done it needs to be done you can't stop it . . . I have thought about it but it doesn't really bother me. [Kate_2_1]

Shown in Helen's account the *fetus* is once again significant around labour. Further, negative images of her baby appear stimulated by *expert* comments. Helen expresses fears that having a big baby will make her labour more painful and different to her expectations, this articulated fear could again be a consequence of the expert labelling of her as an **abnormal pregnant woman**. Once again, however, she devolves responsibility for a potential problem, this time to her partner.

> They've told me it's a big baby so that frightens me a bit. On his side all his side are over 10lbs so that frightens me that it might be a massive baby. It is going to hurt me and that you know is it going to be over real quickly but I can't really say. I just want an average size and over real quick, go in and go out. [Helen_2_2]

Helen's narrative is again reflected in Kate's.

> [I: Do you tend to base your information about the labour that's coming on your past experience?] Yes and no . . . it would be easy if it was like that but you just don't know what to expect do you, like I said this baby's bigger so it might be different. [Kate_2_1]

Women's expectations of labour appear to be constructed from a number of different influences. These narratives suggest that even multigravida women's own **experienced labourer** discourses do not entirely explicate their construction of their expectant labour and for all women *cultural, societal and expert discourse* continue to play a pervasive role.

PROMOTING MOTHERHOOD/RELEGATING FATHERHOOD

Women in late pregnancy have reinforced and rationalised their choices in a slightly different way from early pregnancy. Implicit in their narratives, however, remains the influence of *ideologies of motherhood* by which women measure their performance as **good mothers**. Ownership and responsibility for pregnancy events, choices and decision-making, even when devolved to an extent within the women's accounts, remains their domain. Fathers continue to be situated as *latent fathers* largely absent from decision-making or real involvement with regard to the pregnancy and delivery. Mary's narrative displays that even in late pregnancy women relegate fathers to a latent role. Matt continues to display an obvious emotional connection to the pregnancy but, in contrasting him with herself, Mary still perceives him as incapable of engaging with the reality of pregnancy.

> Erm . . . everything scares him . . . I mean the second the midwife went out the door he just burst into tears . . . he just didn't know what to do, like oh what's happening, what's happening, and I'm saying it's alright, it's alright you know, erm I was fine by that point and I've been absolutely fine through it all really. [Mary_2_2]

Kate supports this, her preference for her mother to be with her at delivery rather than her partner is because of her Mum's ability to understand the labour and birth experience. Kate's partner is relegated to an absent position and not included in this decision-making.

> As long as me Mum's there, don't know I had them both for the first one so as

long as I've got one there for the second. [I: Right, so if you had a choice out of the two?] Mum would be my first choice. [I: Why?] I think cos she's been through it four times and she knows what it's like so. [Kate_2_1]

Sophie's narrative demonstrates her perception that men relegate themselves to a *latent father* role.

Last time I was in labour my Mum and Karl came with me erm . . . he was sort of sat on the sidelines but this time he'll be there with me so they both don't have to come. [Sophie_2_1]

Women's narratives suggest that their expectations of support from their partners are essentially practical. Helen describes her partner as fulfilling the organising role she would normally undertake with regard to the other children, rather than being essential to the labour outcome.

I'd like him to come home, sort the kids out and follow me. [Helen_2_2]

Sophie articulates concerns about how her husband is important in the practicalities of getting to hospital.

[M]y husband is luckily on a course and he's working a different job for a while so he's not going to be on nights but I think what if I went into labour and there's only me and Jack here that's the only thing that worries me a bit what will I do. [Sophie_2_1]

Helen's account goes on to illustrate the fundamental reason she wants her partner present at delivery, despite earlier narratives that articulate his failure to support her in labour. She demonstrates fears of being an **absent mother**. Despite the incidence of maternal mortality being extremely low in this country, the *historical legacy of childbirth*, quite probably reinforced by the *medical discourse*, which has firmly situated Helen as an **abnormal pregnant woman** from an early point in her pregnancy, is inscribed in her mind. Helen needs her partner to be present. Her narrative suggests that she believes birth transforms the *latent father* into *a father* ensuring a parent for the baby if things go wrong in labour.

No as long as I know he's there outside the door, but I think if he was sort of Isle of Wight then I think I'd sort of panic a bit, I'd think what about if this goes wrong, what if that goes wrong, what if I die. [I: Well I'm sure you won't] I know but you never know though do you. [Helen_2_2]

Implicit in women's narratives is that pregnancy, labour and birth remain firmly situated as a female institution. Clearly the *physical experience of pregnancy* plays a fundamental part here. However, it appears that women are actively complicit in keeping fathers to be in this secondary role. The role ascribed to their partners is at worst absent and at best one of support, whilst women are elevated to a role that is fundamental to their babies' survival and requires of them to be **a mother** during pregnancy to ensure a successful outcome.

SUMMARY

Late pregnancy continues to see the *fetus* play an influential role in reinforcing women's **pregnant woman** identity but also it is now attributed with agency in the return to a **non-pregnant woman**. These late pregnancy narratives display the continued and powerful role played by *experts* in the form of doctors and midwives in situating women as **normal pregnant women** or **abnormal pregnant women**. Women firmly locate pregnancy, labour and birth as a female institution, for which they are ultimately accountable. Those women labelled as abnormal and positioned as **maternity patients** find their personal ownership of the pregnancy weakened as control over the pregnancy is ceded to the *experts* and choice is removed. Women are ultimately complicit with this in order to maintain their **good mother** status. Expectations of labour narratives demonstrate the continued and significant influence of societal and cultural discourses in illuminating the choices women made in early pregnancy and further illustrate how women strive to promote themselves as **good mothers**.

REFERENCES

1 Gatrell C. *Hard Labour: the sociology of parenthood.* Maidenhead: Open University Press; 2005.

2 Oakley A. *Essays on Women, Medicine and Health.* Edinburgh: Edinburgh University Press; 1993.

CHAPTER 7

So how was it? Giving birth and the early postnatal days

2–4 WEEKS AFTER BIRTH

A third set of interviews took place following delivery, when women generally related their labour and perinatal stories. Characters revealed in earlier narratives, such as *experts*, as well as narrative identities, such as **good mother/bad mother** and **maternity patients**, continue to infuse the themes that arise. These appear alongside other characters and identities, which have replaced or evolved from those identified earlier.

The following themes evolved but remained from pregnancy:

➤ experts and expertise: being a maternity patient
➤ promoting motherhood/relegating fatherhood.

The new themes apparent in the early postnatal period include:

➤ fetal role in labour
➤ birth creates real mothers.

EXPERTS AND EXPERTISE: BEING A MATERNITY PATIENT

Women's late pregnancy narratives illustrated how women, such as Polly, indirectly situated themselves as **maternity patients** through deference to *experts* to affirm the status of their pregnancies. For others, such as Mary, the *physical symptoms of pregnancy* located her as an **abnormal pregnant woman** and through subsequent monitoring by *experts* as a **maternity patient**. For most women in late pregnancy, however, a **maternity patient** identity did not feature and in Helen's case was firmly resisted. Narratives following delivery saw most women articulate some loss of control or choice and emergence of a **maternity patient** identity, irrespective of their original choices for delivery.

In Mary's late-pregnancy accounts, raised blood pressure situated her as a **maternity patient**; devolved not unwillingly, as shown in those narratives, of personal control over events relating to her pregnancy. Mary as **abnormal pregnant woman** was placed under the control of *medical experts* to assure her well-being and that of her baby.

> I was about 38 weeks and I went in and my diastolic was 110 again on the tablets so she said, and I'd really blown up you know like you really do and one thing and another and erm the bloods that they took that day were starting to really show so they got me in to induce me so when they monitored me they said they think you're in early labour anyway . . . so they let me go on and I got through to about midnight I think and erm . . . and my blood pressure went sky high absolutely . . . so they said we can't mess about now so they said we'll put a pessary . . . and then I got to about 3–4cm then they broke my waters and erm then started. I'd had an epidural for when they started me on a drip as well and they'd wanted me to have an epidural for my blood pressure so I'd been getting ready for it . . . I went all through the day and erm they were monitoring all afternoon because of my blood pressure and I was absolutely fast asleep and I woke up really suddenly and I just knew, it was so really weird and I looked and it (baby's heartbeat) was really dipped on the monitor and the nurse was there and within half an hour they had me in for a caesarean. [Mary_3_1]

This post-delivery account demonstrates the language used by the *experts* as her pregnancy progresses, suggesting urgency and potential danger, which only they as *experts* have the knowledge and skill to manage. Mary as shown is completely disempowered by the chain of events but relates this as a heroic tale. The *experts* allowed her a chance to labour and she 'messed about', conferring her with a **failed woman** identity, unable to independently conclude her pregnancy when necessary. Hence *experts* who have greater knowledge and expertise step in. Mary, as a consequence of her **maternity patient** identity and the need to maintain her **good mother** status, acting to ensure her baby's well-being readily and unquestioningly accepts interventions such as induction and an epidural. She earnestly articulates, however, her own personal contribution to maintaining and asserting her **good mother** identity. Claims that she was in spontaneous labour signify that despite her location by *experts* as a **failed woman**, she had an innate reaction to the intrinsic danger, which initiated action. Mary's account further suggests that her construction as an **abnormal pregnant woman** albeit through events beyond her control requires her to compensate for being a **bad**

mother, who has failed to maintain a normal healthy pregnancy, affecting her body and consequently her baby. This is reinforced in the above narrative when she demonstrates herself as a **good mother** through her innate sense of her baby's well-being. The fetal monitor provides technological confirmation of her **good mother** identity. Mary above demonstrates no fear for the ramifications on her own health, emphasising further the self-sacrificing act of a **good mother**. Mary in her narrative is unquestioning of the expert decisions and the necessity of intervention. It seems reasonable to suggest that this is a consequence of her rationale for her choice of site for delivery, expressed in both her early and late pregnancy narratives. Despite desires articulated in late pregnancy for a normal delivery the expectation of problems was ever present and resulted in a pragmatic attitude to pregnancy and labour.

Jane's narrative will be explored in some detail in this section, because of its direct relevance to the theme. In contrast to Mary, as was shown in early and late pregnancy narratives, Jane articulates a desire for a non-medical, non-interventionalist approach to her delivery and here reinforces her rationale for choosing a birth-centre delivery. Her suggestion that the main unit is associated with trauma conflicts with *culturally commodified notions of birth* as normal and natural,[1] which Jane appears to desire and the birth centre as a 'home from home' environment, appears to support. This narrative below suggests that the ability to act independently and maintain control resists a **maternity patient** identity and promotes the image of a relaxed and **controlled labourer** that women's narratives in late pregnancy demonstrated as important.

> I don't like hospitals and obviously the main unit has got a very hospital atmosphere and that the birthing centre is just like being at home so you can walk about when you wanted you can go and make your own drinks and things like that so I just liked the whole atmosphere, the fact that it was so relaxed, and I liked the birthing pool, I mean I know they've got a birthing pool at the main unit as well but I just liked the whole atmosphere but all in all I think it's that it's more like being at home and a bit less traumatic than being hospital but. [Jane_3_2]

Jane's story continued below shows that despite a very clear preference for the type of environment and experience desired, pregnancy related events resulted in a removal of choice and transfer to the acute unit for delivery.

> Horrific [crying], no it wasn't horrific I'm been melodramatic there but it just didn't go to plan erm . . . my waters broke on the Friday morning and nothing else happened erm so we went up to the birth centre . . . nothing still had

happened so they went through the . . . if you want it up there then 72 hours is the limit, they like them out before 72 hours don't they so they said we need something to be happening shortly, so the sent me off sent me off home, I kept having contractions on and off . . . by Sunday afternoon, 3.00, I was only 3 cm. [I: were you contracting though?] Yeah I was contracting but nothing opening so she said I'm sorry you're gonna have to go [to the main unit] . . . we're running out of hours now to get him out, so they put me on a drip and obviously they're monitoring him and monitoring me and then I obviously had the gas and air but time was banging on and the consultant had said that I might have to have a caesarean because it still wasn't but the midwives were excellent up there and they said look you really should . . . [I: was this the midwives at the main unit then?] At the main unit yeah, they were absolutely fantastic for all my reservations about actually going up there and being left I had two . . . and one was with me all the way through and they said look to relax you we suggest you have an epidural and that was the worst thing the thing I really did not want an epidural at all, so they said its either that or caesarean really because we need to get you fully dilated and I thought well I don't want to be laid up for so I thought well . . . lesser of two evils and I felt fantastic and I thought why didn't I have one of these to begin with [laughs] but there you go but then I slept for a while and by the time I'd woken up I was 9 cm so there you go. [Jane_3_2]

Professional guidelines are utilised here as the mouthpiece of *experts* acting under the remit of ensuring a safe and healthy delivery outcome and prevent Jane from remaining at the birth centre. Jane becomes labelled as an **abnormal pregnant woman** under the remit of *medical experts* and thus relegated to the status of **maternity patient**, on a drip being monitored, placid, compliant and disempowered. There is an acknowledgement that the hospitalised experience was not as bad as envisaged. However the removal of control and choice conflicts with Jane's idealised notions of birth and is a significant emotional experience apparent in these early postnatal narratives. The *experts*, as for Mary, play a fundamental role in locating Jane as a **failed woman**, stating 'we need something to be happening shortly' suggesting that the responsibility for becoming an **abnormal pregnant women** by failing to go into labour is Jane's. This can be read as a transference of responsibility for failure to fulfil the promise of choice from the *experts* and the system and directly on to the woman. Clear reference to the safety of the baby based on *expert knowing* means failure to comply would indicate irresponsibility and construct Jane as a **bad mother**. Jane clearly demonstrates the dominance of her **good mother** identity, despite her obvious distress she prioritises the well-being of her baby and diminishes the importance of personal choice and experience.

[T]he most important thing was him and there would have been no questions about it, but he was fine . . . I'm alright now. [Jane_3_2]

Mary also demonstrates how women rank their baby's well-being above their own personal desires and satisfaction with their birth experience.

I don't think you can, I think its erm I don't know that anything can prepare you for it really, like you say if not perhaps the best experience in the world and the rush down to theatre, you still get that feeling, it seems to make all that seem quite irrelevant. [Mary_3_1]

Unlike Mary who does not differentiate *experts* in her above narrative, referring to 'they', there is a clear separation of the experts in Jane's narrative between *midwife experts* and consultants as *medical experts*. Jane and Mary present converse narratives about who is afforded the more significant *expert* role in their labours. For Mary it is the doctors; this is implicit in her acceptance of her **maternity patient** identity.

You just go with the flow and have complete confidence with everything, what everyone was doing, I mean the staff were great, the doctors were lovely. [Mary_3_1]

Jane, despite having been situated as a **maternity patient**, clings to her *idealised notions of labour* and desire for a normal delivery and credits the midwives with supporting her resistance against a **maternity patient** identity.

No, no I did think I might have ended up with one (a caesarean) but no the midwives said no we'll get him out, no I mean they were excellent considering the consultant kept coming in and wanting me to go for a caesarean and they were like you've really got to start pushing now I had sort of resigned myself to the fact that well it would be so much easier if I had a caesarean and they were like Jane you don't need this you can deliver naturally, you're not gonna need one and we're gonna make sure and that encouraged me a bit but there were times when I just thought oh for gods sake just get him out, if she'd come in again I probably would have said yes but the midwives were like no you're going to do it, I'll keep telling her that you're getting there you're getting there but there were times when I thought it was the best option. [Jane_3_2]

Apparent in both narratives is how decision-making choice and personal control was completely removed by the *experts*, but is articulated as a positive action and as good care in light of a successful labour outcome. Polly and Sally's narratives also demonstrate that removal of personal control is not perceived as a negative action, supporting the argument that more important to many women than direct control is personal control over when to relinquish control.[2,3]

> That last stage of pushing was the hardest when I really didn't think I had it in me but fortunately, the midwife who was supervising the ward came in and gave me that sharp shock treatment I needed and she was born at 5.25. [Polly_3_1]

> [I]t was ventouse in the end . . . they just wanted to get it I wasn't bothered by that time because I was tired and I just wanted her out. [Sally_3_1]

Helen's labour account echoes the fears she articulated in both early and late pregnancy about delivering without *expert* input. Premature labour confirmed Helen's suspected status as an **abnormal pregnant woman** and necessitated delivery at the acute unit as a **maternity patient**, which she had tried to avoid.

> Well, it was very quick, I expected to be early and I was . . . we organised the kids and went to the hospital . . . I arrived about 3.10 and she was born at 3.47. [I: Not much time then, how did you feel?] Very panicky that I wasn't going to be there in time. [Helen_3_1]

Her labour, concordant with the expectations expressed in pregnancy, is a negative one. Although she does not refer to a lack of personal control, it seems implicit in her narrative that her desire to have been a **controlled labourer**, which she believed would have been facilitated by delivery at the nearer birth centre, is unfulfilled.

> Horrible, horrible the pain was horrible and I only had time for gas and air, it was the worst of all three, the contractions were really painful and the pushing erm . . . the crowning was awful really painful, I don't know why but it was the worst of all three of them. [Helen_3_1]

One of the apparent difficulties in offering women choice in maternity care appears to be the powerful role that *experts* play in locating women as **maternity patients** when it conflicts with women's personal desires. Jane, Helen and Kate all articulate the emotional consequences of a negative birth experience, which situated them as **maternity patients** and devolved them of choice and control.

[M]y midwife said, she said 'if you could have second babies first then there would be no problems, I think it's just the unknown as well, as I said I don't think you're prepared and if someone had told me it was going to be like that I don't know whether I'd have done it, I don't think I would have had kids at all . . . People say that, that you'll forget but I won't, I won't forget. [Jane_3_2]

No I'm getting sterilised . . . I'm on the waiting list. [Helen_3_1]

No my labour wasn't as long, but it was painful though . . . never again, that's it now . . . that's finished me, it wouldn't have been so bad if it had happened straight away, it was 2 hours after they got it in (the drip). [Kate_3_1]

An interesting aspect of this particular theme is that the women interviewed who were constructed as **normal pregnant women** and maintained that status throughout labour, tended to narrate extremely positive birth experiences. Even in those circumstances, however, some narratives display the role *experts* play in influencing women's labour events and choices, as in Julie's account below with regard to an epidural.

I mean they were just absolutely fantastic . . . I had two really young midwives and they never left me all night she was rubbing my back, she got me the birthing ball . . . the midwife just stood and watched me if I wanted my back rubbing she'd rub my back for me, it was only in the early hours of the morning when I wanted some pain relief and I wanted to know how I was doing and she said 'shall we just look and see how you're doing' and she examined me and my waters still hadn't gone . . . she said 'your waters are bulging' and I was five centimetres dilated . . . I was absolutely shattered so I said I want an epidural but they seemed reluctant to give you the epidural, you know 'once you have an epidural then things can go wrong you know, what about pethidine' so she gave me the pethidine which just helped me to rest in between contractions [I: just took the edge of] then she just gave me some gas and air . . . then I said I wanted something else and they talked me into having Meptid but that did absolutely nothing . . . and when that did nothing I demanded an epidural so the midwife went to get the anaesthetist who was in theatre . . . by the time he came back with his mate she was at the foot of the bed . . . just three pushes and she was out, so I was glad at the end of it I didn't have an epidural. [Julie_3_1]

In contrast to Julie, Sally demanded an epidural and was given one. Sally narrates the midwives role as an *expert* in situating her as a **normal pregnant woman**, which despite medical intervention in the form of an epidural left her feeling she had retained personal control over choice and decision-making in labour.

I think I had two lots of pethidine and I sat on the birthing ball, I was going to go for a water birth but when I sat in the bath and it was so painful I thought no I don't think so. [I: So you decided not to?] Yeah so I spoke to the girl and said I wanted an epidural and the anaesthetist was in theatre so she said she'd book me in for the next slot and within half an hour that was in and as soon when I got the epidural it was brilliant just enjoyable really . . . I don't think it was too bad, I was quite pleased with that . . . the midwife was fantastic . . . she was just great . . . she stayed with me all the time. [Sally_3_1]

This theme illustrates two key concepts. Firstly that women may have *commodified ideas of childbirth* that are overridden not only by labour events but by the physical pain of childbirth, which renders them out of control. More importantly, however, it highlights the role that *experts* play in locating women as **maternity patients**. Women's narratives demonstrate the disempowering consequences of being given this identity in labour. For women like Mary who made original choices influenced by *medical discourse* this was accepted and even praised. For others who wanted a normal and natural experience the emotional distress is apparent. It seems that there may be inherent consequences in offering choice and failing to fulfil that choice, which may be more emotionally damaging to women than if choice did not exist.

THE FETAL ROLE IN LABOUR

Helen's accounts in late pregnancy afforded the *fetus* a clear role with regard to labour, and these post-delivery narratives clearly echo that sentiment. Most women now ascribe the *fetus* agency and an active role in labour. Mary describes how her caesarean delivery was due to her baby's position, which was not conducive to a normal delivery.

[T]hey were going to try and use forceps but he was brow presentation as well and it was still really high up so they said it would have made a mess of him and was a bit messy for me and upsetting even more. [Mary_3_1]

Sally's account also supports an active role for the *fetus* in dictating labour interventions and outcomes.

[H]er heartbeat was up and down normally they would have let me do it but with her heart beat out was up and down they just wanted to get it. [Sally_3_1]

Jane attributes her *fetus* with a responsibility for getting into the wrong position and prolonging her labour.

> [U]nfortunately he was the wrong, his back was to my back so erm so it was a long drawn out because they were trying to turn him I think but he came eventually. [Jane_3_2]

The *fetus* throughout pregnancy is afforded a powerful role in influencing women's choices, decision and events. Despite the dependant status of the *fetus* up to the point of delivery, which women clearly recognise, personhood is conferred on the *fetus* particularly with regard to labour narratives where it is ascribed a very active role in determining events. This clearly merits further interpretation, particularly as we saw the difficulties some women had in late pregnancy in visualising their babies as real. The language used in these accounts could provide one explanation. Women refer to their babies as he or she, which for many women remains unknown until after delivery. It seems feasible to suggest that when women narrate their labour experience it inevitably incorporates and reflects the developing relationships with their babies in the early postnatal period. This allows them to visualise their babies not only by gender but also as individuals within their labour experience and attributes them a clear role.

BABIES CREATE 'REAL MOTHERS'

Pregnancy has seen the role played by the *fetus* in creating **mothers** and the dichotomous **good mother/bad mother** identity as women take on characteristics of the mothering role. Above we have also seen the fetus being ascribed human characteristics in labour. Following the *birth of the baby*, the baby becomes an actual character within the story with its own individuality, rather than the proxy character with agency that existed for women in pregnancy. The *birth of the baby* formally facilitates societal and personal recognition of the woman as **a real mother**. The *fetus* during pregnancy, compelled women to aspire to a **good mother** identity, depicted by *ideologies of mothering*. Women's early post-delivery narratives suggest that their mothering, although aspiring to the same ideology, takes on a different content from that apparent in pregnancy.

In late pregnancy, Mary narrated as elusive an emotional connection to her *fetus* promoting her fears of being a **bad mother**. This account of her response to the birth fills the emotional gap, meets the *cultural depictions of maternal response to birth*[4] and captures that emotional connection affirming her as both 'a real mother' and a **good mother**.

> [I]t's so much more emotional and you do love them so much don't you, it
> just bowled me over, you know the whole emotional experience just bowled
> me over, yeah it's wonderful, it's amazing the sort of things you go through . . .
> nothing prepares you for. [Mary_3_1]

Jane who worried, in pregnancy, about her lack of experience with children
and so also feared being a **bad mother** describes how following birth she is **a
real mother** with an innate mothering ability and sense of how to care for her
own son.

> [O]bviously it has changed my life but I think although I'm not particularly
> maternal with other peoples children I was thinking what will I be like with my
> own and even simple things like just picking him up and simple things I was
> thinking but him I'm not you feel just so its just so easy. [Jane_3_2]

Polly supports the emotional response that accompanies the *birth of the baby*
but in addition recognises that **a real mother** identity brings with it a reality of
mothering that did not exist before birth.

> [Y]ou feel completely elated because you've got this tiny miracle laid in your
> arms and you can't believe that you've been carrying that for 9 months and
> suddenly it's real. [Polly_3_1]

Sally further supports how the mothering role she played in pregnancy does not
carry the same demands as being **a real mother** and articulates a reality that
is different to the expectations depicted by *romantic notions of motherhood* as a
wonderful and fulfilling experience for women.[5]

> She dictates everything you do, if we go out it's when she says and I didn't really
> expect it. [Sally_3_1]

Helen's story illustrates how being **a real mother**, brings to reality the emotional
dimensions that were intangible for some women in pregnancy.

> OK at first but then pretty horrible. [I: why?] Well she [baby] got jaundice and
> had to go in HRI, [I: oh no] they were brilliant there though, I stayed all the
> time, she had to have phototherapy and they gave her a drip . . . it was horrible
> I really thought she was dying. [Helen_3_1]

The **bad mother** identity, revealed in women's narratives during pregnancy, based on fears that their physical state, actions and decisions might be linked to bad pregnancy outcomes, is now created by an inescapable reality of visible events and outcomes. An *unhealthy/abnormal baby*, as in pregnancy, can signify a failure to nurture and protect. The fear narrated by Helen here is consistent with that articulated in the pregnancy narratives but the strong emotional connection with the baby is apparent, generated by the reality of *the birth of the baby*, creating Helen's status as **a real mother** who loves her baby. Her failure, however, is now visible and can be directly attributed to her bad decisions and failure to notice a problem. Her narrative below demonstrates both intrinsic feelings of guilt and failure, and how her **bad mother** identity is reinforced by the blame afforded by others.

> Really upset and I just wanted to cry all the time erm . . . I just didn't really know what to make of it and he (husband) thought it was my fault because I wanted to come home quickly and I didn't need that. . . . I said 'she's been examined and they said everything was OK' so you believe that don't you? I was worried that it was my fault anyway and he just made it worse . . . You just assume the worst don't you [I: mmm] I really did think the worst when she was ill. [Helen_3_1]

As women did in pregnancy, Helen is quick to try and reinstate her **good mother** identity by describing her actions when her daughter was ill. Helen narrates the characteristics of a **good mother**; i.e. responsibility, advocacy and a self-sacrificing relegation of her own personal needs. She reinforces herself as a **good mother** by contrasting her behaviour to that of other **bad mothers**.

> I couldn't sleep I was listening all the time for her and I didn't dare leave her . . . some parents left their kids I can't understand it, one day I came home for a shower and to get some clean clothes and try and get a bit of rest but I felt really guilty leaving her even for two hours in case something happened erm . . . [Helen_3_1]

Mary, Sally and Jane tell less dramatic accounts but still go on to further describe the physical realities of being **a real mother** that make demands beyond those that mothering in pregnancy requires.

> It is hard work, you're just constantly on the ball aren't you . . . I think it's true that your life totally changes. [Jane_3_2]

Sally again shows how being **a real mother** fails to meet *romantic notions of* *motherhood* and how that leaves her feeling unprepared and alone. There is both a physical recovery and emotional adjustment taking place in Sally's narrative that is clearly traumatic.

> Mixed emotions really . . . nothing can prepare you for it, nothing at all obviously been a bit tired because I've lost so much blood but I've been a bit weepy as well and obviously then he went away and I was like 'thanks a lot she's only two weeks old' . . . and suddenly when he went away it was like 'oh I've got to do this on my own' . . . I think as well I never get a break. [Sally_3_1]

Mary also narrates about tiredness, which she acknowledges impacts on the emotional adjustment to being **a real mother**, which contrasts sharply with the earlier euphoria.

> I was just on a high for about 2 weeks and then probably about a week ago I got a bit of a 'oh heck', I was tired, I was really tired and thinking oh no, I'll never get a decent nights sleep . . . and the thing is if I get tired everything goes down with me my mood goes I don't seem to be able to get on with it really and the first sign of me not feeling happy and that sounds awful because I've got this baby and I should be over the moon but I wasn't at all I was tired and fed up and he was crying and I probably had sore nipples too and he wasn't latching on properly. [Mary_3_1]

Mary as **a real mother** provides emotional narratives that display a sense of shock, frustration and overwhelming responsibility, and also seem to hint at some loss of personal identity as identified in other work on the transition to motherhood.[1,6] She is, however, quick to assert her **good mother** identity with claims that motherhood is *lovely really*.

> Its 24 hours isn't it and as you know, there's no break from it, you don't get a couple of days off, its always thinking of them, what they need, what the matter and the fact they can't tell you things and they're utterly in your hands and if things go wrong you sort of feel as if its your fault really but erh lovely really. [Mary_3_1]

What all these narrative show is that the *birth of the baby* creates **a real mother**, an identity that incorporates many of the characteristics aspired to in pregnancy, including nurturing, advocacy, protection, responsibility for a dependant that relies almost exclusively on the biological mother, being self-sacrificing and accountable. However, **a real mother** created by the *birth of the baby* demands from women a totally child-centred approach and contains the emotional involvement that was lacking for women in pregnancy. These women's accounts suggest that mothering following birth is a significantly more physically- and emotionally-demanding role than mothering performed when pregnant, and women's adaptation to **a real mother** role appears to be affected by their expectations, physical recovery from labour and post-delivery events.

PROMOTING MOTHERHOOD/RELEGATING FATHERHOOD

As the pregnancy test hails the woman as **pregnant woman**, so *the birth of the baby* hails her as **a real mother**. There is recognition that *the birth of the baby* creates a new type of mothering, creating an identity different in mothering content to before birth. Women who in pregnancy have relegated their partners to a *latent father* status, following delivery now articulate a perception of their partners that affords them a *fathering* role. Their partners are clearly characters within the story and fathers in concrete terms, however, women still construct their partners as *a father* in a certain way that is an extension of the pregnancy construction; this continues to afford women a higher parenting status with regard to their baby than their partners. Helen's narrative below supports traditional *gendered parenting discourses*, situating her husband as simply less capable than her, but more importantly unable to be self-sacrificing and relegate his needs as secondary to the children in the way that mothers are expected to be. She further suggests that despite the inherent difficulties of being **a real mother** she has no option, because to shirk the responsibility would render her a **bad mother**, whilst she perceives that as *a father* he retains an opt-out clause, which does not categorise him as a *bad father*.

> He had to look after the kids whilst I was in hospital with her and he realised how hard it is to look after the kids, do the housework, make sure they do all their homework and everything . . . he actually said to me he realised that its hard to be a woman and he didn't realise how much there actually was to do . . . He feels neglected, he's complaining all the time that there's no time for him so I said 'there's no time for myself never mind you' he just makes me cross . . . he just doesn't see all the things I have to do, I know women can multi-task but there's a limit. [Helen_3_1]

Jane supports the depiction of the man as less culturally bound to his new role as *a father* than hers as **a mother**, even though parenthood was wanted by them both and considered a joint venture. Jane's need to assert her **good mother** identity remains consistent in her claims that she 'wouldn't have it any other way', and that her mothering is successful. Her story, however, also highlights the pressure that *gendered parenting discourses* exert on women to unquestioningly behave in a way that conforms to the gendered depiction of mothers.

> I think it's true that your life totally changes and theirs doesn't, I mean Paul does a lot of climbing and he's still out, I mean I wouldn't stop him going unless I felt really below par he wouldn't go, but no he goes out to football on a Monday night and he still goes climbing for 2 hours, whereas the best I get is nipping down the shop in between feeds . . . and you just think gosh your life is just you know . . . I just feel like a big feeding machine you know but I wouldn't have it any other way, he's very content and very healthy but . . . [Jane_3_2]

Sally supports Helen in suggesting that as *a father*, her partner's sense of responsibility and innate understanding of the baby's needs is simply not as strong as hers. Her narrative goes further than Jane's in questioning the fairness of imposed *gendered parenting roles*.

> [H]is life hasn't changed and yours has changed completely, I haven't said anything but I do think 'its not fair, you know its not fair I mean he'll help out a bed time and that which is nice but he's not I'm always with her totally throughout the day . . . trying to get him to see she was crying yesterday and he just put her in her pram and left her and I said 'you can't just leave her crying' and he said 'you can't pick her up all the time' and I said 'yeah but she's been crying quite a long time' and he can do that he can cut off from her or whatever but I can't leave her to cry I can do it for so long but then I have to pick her up and check she's alright . . . and than I get mad because things have changed and he's got to be different and I see that. He can go away and have a bit of a break and adult conversations and I get a bit you know . . . [Sally_3_1]

Kate supports the concept of an 'opt-out clause' for fathers in narrating how fatherhood for her partner, because they are separated, does not carry the same intrinsic responsibilities that motherhood carries. Kate's role as **a real mother** involves an inescapable responsibility for the baby despite the end of an intimate relationship.

> I was worried about how I would manage, but his dad hasn't seen him, I just don't know when or if he'll get over . . . [Kate_3_1]

Mary goes on to demonstrate that significant influence that the *institution of motherhood* plays in defining the designated roles that denote **good mothers**.

She shows the personal emotional impact that responsibility carries when women feel they are failing and are **bad mothers**.

> [H]e was screaming he was obviously hungry and I just couldn't get him on I couldn't get me head around it and I couldn't think and I was just crying. I'm just not being a very good Mum . . . the responsibility overwhelms me a little bit. [Mary_3_1]

Polly here narrates the responsibility for the baby as hers, underpinned by a fear of being a **bad mother**, with no reference to her partner at all. There seems, as with Mary earlier, an implicit loss of personal identity, that of a person in control who existed prior to the *birth of the baby*.

> I've got to admit the first three weeks I've been absolutely petrified to the point where I've felt like a frightened little child . . . I like to be in control and to all of a sudden have this massive responsibility and not really know what to do with it because you've never experienced it before I found quite overwhelming. [Polly_3_1]

Midwife experts as Polly's story continues, go on to exacerbate a **bad mother** identity. The midwives create an identity where a **good mother** chooses to breastfeed and is successful at it and Polly's failure to achieve this locates her as a **bad mother** and a failure.

> I wanted to be the best mother I could and by not achieving the breastfeeding aspects I was actually failing . . . the other things are insignificant, the nappy changing the bathing, etc. but the breast feeding is such a big issue and the midwives and everything leading up to it in your pregnancy give such an importance to breastfeeding . . . but when it's not happening it makes you feel you're failing. [Polly_3_1]

Polly accepts total responsibility for feeding choices and so her guilt and feelings of failure are personal. Her partner is sidelined and located as someone who is unable to engage with or understand a prioritising of the baby's well-being over Polly's own.

> You completely change once you've had that baby and anybody like James saying don't worry it's (breastfeeding) not a matter of life and death, it was to me. [Polly_3_1]

Helen reinforces how being a **good mother** is inexorable and linked to her baby's very survival.

> I just wanted to do what was best for her; I really did think the worst when she was ill, I thought she was going to die. [Helen_3_1]

There are *culturally mediated standards* of the *institution of motherhood* to adhere to and things to do right that depict a **good mother**. There is importance attached to coping, even though her partner is present as *a father* and undertaking child-care tasks. Rob, is actually depicted below, as being detrimental to the organised family environment. This might suggest that the relegation of fatherhood is actually fundamental to women in promoting their status as a **good mother**.

> Before she was born I had everything done be a certain time . . . so it was getting to half past twelve and I wasn't dressed and Amelia wasn't dressed, I'm tripping over Rob, he's doing bottles, it was just organised chaos and I'm thinking I'm never gonna get the hang of this . . . I was saying I can't cope and I'm not doing it right. [Julie_3_1]

The *ideologies of mothering* and the *institution of motherhood* set the cultural and societal standards that women strive for as **a real mother**. These standards invest women with a *gendered parenting role* and a fundamental responsibility for their children; such a responsibility is absent from their perceptions of fathering. Despite contemporary notions of parenthood as a joint venture, in which both parents have responsibility, in their narratives women remain constrained by the societal norms of themselves as both the natural and default carer, and are complicit in relegating their partners to the traditional support and back-up role.

Societal expectations have a powerful effect on women; whilst they strive to achieve traditional depictions of a **good mother** constrained by *culturally mediated standards of motherhood*, complexity is added by *contemporary notions of fathers* as active parents. In some narratives women locate themselves as part of a fulfilled and loving family, based on cultural and media depictions of *an ideal modern family life*. References to bonding depict a father investing in an emotional relationship with his baby, in contrast to the previous depictions of him as simply less involved and responsible.

> Matt and I felt a need to bond together as a family . . . you need to don't you, to get to know him first. [Mary_3_1]

> I wanted us all to bond together. [Julie_3_1]

The experience of being **a real mother** for women is physically and emotionally demanding. In addition there is a suggestion that women feel they are only **a mother** and unable to be what they were before birth. A *father* in general is not perceived as having to adhere to equivalent standards or make the same life changes. This depiction of the fathers as less involved, less responsible and less engaged in their roles is an apparent extension of the role women allocate their partners from early pregnancy.

SUMMARY

Early postnatal narratives, which reflected on labour, emphasise the powerful role that *experts* play during women's labour experiences in depriving them of control and choice. The continued aspiration to be a **good mother** disempowers women in labour and reinforces *expert* power. Moreover the language used by experts suggests that it is women's own inadequate labouring performances that are responsible for any loss of choice and control. The emotional ramifications for some women of being located as a **maternity patient** and robbed of the desired birth experience promised through choice are apparent. Consumerist discourse offers women access to *commodified notions of birth* as normal and natural whilst *the medical discourse* retains the authority to override such aspirations. Whilst women have performed a form of mothering during pregnancy the reality of mothering following birth is narrated as both different in content and as a shock to women in this early postnatal period. The powerful role that societal discourses around *parenting* and *traditional gendered roles* play is inherently forceful in women's adaptation to a **real mother** role.

REFERENCES

1 Gatrell C. *Hard Labour: the sociology of parenthood.* Maidenhead: Open University Press; 2005.
2 Weaver J. Childbirth. In: Ussher JM, editor. *Women's Health: contemporary international health perspectives.* Leicester: The British Psychological Society; 2000.
3 Green J, Baston H. Feeling in control during labour: concepts, correlates and consequences. *Birth.* 2003; **30**(4): 235–47.
4 Kitzinger S. *Ourselves as Mothers.* London: Doubleday; 1992.
5 Woollett A, Marshall H. Motherhood and mothering. In: Ussher JM, editor. *Women's Health: contemporary international health perspectives.* Leicester: The British Psychological Society; 2000.
6 Oakley A. *From Here to Maternity: becoming a mother.* Harmondsworth: Penguin; 1981.

CHAPTER 8

'No going back': the reality of mothering

SIX MONTHS POSTNATAL

The fourth interviews took place six months after the women had given birth. In this late postnatal period, the **good mother/bad mother** dichotomy still remains a consistent identity for women. Many of the discourses and influences present from pregnancy including *experts, ideologies of motherhood*, and *idealised notions of birth* can still be seen, though the women articulate them differently by this time. One theme remains consistent with earlier findings:

➤ experts and expertise.

The new themes evident include:

➤ reflecting on labour
➤ choice and satisfaction
➤ what about postnatal choice?
➤ maternity experience, choice and postnatal depression.

As in earlier findings Helen and Mary's narratives will feature strongly, with quotes from other women being used to illustrate the themes identified.

REFLECTING ON LABOUR

Women's reflection on their birth experience tended to be much shorter, more general and less graphic than in their early postnatal narratives, and reflect a more positive story of labour than in the early postnatal period as in Helen's account.

> No, no, I'm just glad it was a quick one, not a long drawn-out thing. I was quite happy with a nice quick one, I don't think I could be 24 hours and I can't stand pain but I expected it to be quick though, I expected to be early and I expected to be quick and I was. [Helen_4_1]

Some women's memories are not reflective of actual events, but are consistent with their early postnatal accounts, which situate labour as a positive experience. Others, however, who were negative in the early postnatal days continue to remember labour in negative terms. Polly is typical of the first group of women. During this interview she focussed on feelings rather than the experience of labour itself. In addition, she reinforces the idea of an idealised experience 'it was almost like a textbook pregnancy and birth'.

> It was such a nice experience and it was enjoyable really all the way through, I was never in any real discomfort I remember everything as if was . . . all the memories I have are nice and pleasurable and I wouldn't hesitate to go through them again . . . everything went smoothly and it was almost like a textbook pregnancy and birth. [Polly_4_1]

Jane typifies the second group of women; again there is a focus on feelings and a refusal to recount the actual experience of labour. These feelings clearly inform her intentions not to have any more children.

> Yeah I'm over it now, it's still upsetting but I'm still not planning another one . . . we don't dwell on it. [Jane_4_1]

Sophie's account of her disappointing labour experience is like Jane and Polly's, devoid of any detail, but reflects the ramifications of unfulfilled choice.

> I was going to write a letter to complain, I just think I can't be bothered . . . it was bad at the time . . . I think if I'd known that I could have gone through it without an epidural which is the only reason why I went to the main unit I would have preferred to have gone to the birth centre it sounds a lot more chilled out and you get a lot more better care but you can't undo it now. [Sophie _4_1]

EXPERTS AND EXPERTISE

Despite the comparative brevity of these accounts at this stage, *experts* remain an essential aspect of the women's labour experiences. In Sophie's account (above), she is suggesting that choices for site of birth are made on judgements of available expertise. Failure to be able to access the type of expertise that informed her choice leads to dissatisfaction with her experience. Mary here, as early post-delivery, does not question *expert's* decisions and advice. Here we see the continued promotion of her **good mother** status as she stresses her contribution towards spontaneous labour.

> Gosh it's much harder to remember now, they were monitoring my blood pressure anyway, and they sent me in because it was high and decided to induce me, I had some prostaglandin and I think about 12ish they came to break my waters but they thought I was going into labour myself. Then about 9.00 I was starting to get some pains. I coped quite well I thought then a bit later the pains were starting to get a lot stronger and the midwife came in and suggested an epidural because the anaesthetist was going into theatre and it might be a while before I could have one, so I did. [Mary_4_1]

Mary's narrative depicts her as willingly relinquishing control of decision-making in labour. A feasible proposition is that offering choices for maternity care has failed to facilitate a fundamental shift in power from *experts* to women in labour. Midwives and doctors are often not clearly differentiated and both hold powerful, if slightly differing, roles as *experts*. Hence, women question their own innate sense of their bodies (*personal knowing*) and consequently their judgement and their choices. Mary was devolved of decision-making and personal control by midwives with regard to pain relief in labour, *expert knowing* was accepted as superior and overruled *personal knowing*.

> I was glad she suggested it really, because the pains were getting much worse, I was coping but didn't think I would for much longer. I didn't know when to ask for pain relief, I didn't know whether the pains were really bad or whether I just wasn't coping and I didn't want to seem like a wimp, I mean I'd asked for gas and air earlier on and they said 'oh no you don't want that' so I sort of thought 'oh I must seem like a right wimp'. Also they were going to start Syntocinon and she said the pains would get really bad. [Mary_4_1]

This earlier removal of power and decision-making created an environment in which Mary felt unable to articulate her personal choice with regard to delivery preference.

> The doctor came in and examined me and I'd got to 10 centimetres and Josh was face down so he said that he could do a high forceps, which was the only

> thing I really didn't want, or a section, I thought 'I wish they'd just go for a section because I really didn't want a forceps delivery anyway he came back and he said he'd spoken to the consultant and that he said to go straight for a section and that was it . . . [I: Did you say you would have preferred a section?] No, no I didn't. [Mary_4_1]

Jane equally did not feel able to question an unwanted intervention based on expert advise to ensure the safe delivery of her baby. She also displays her **good mother** identity in the self-sacrificing of her own personal satisfaction for her baby's well-being.

> Yeah that's it at one point I thought I was going to have to have a caesarean and that was another thing I just didn't want but at the end of the day it doesn't matter what more important is that he just comes out okay. [Jane_4_1]

Models for choice assume that women feel able to exercise their rights and make choices when in fact they remain constrained by the belief that *experts* know best and to question that knowledge may well result in detrimental outcomes, which can then be directly attributed to the women themselves as **bad mothers**. What has remained consistent throughout is that women prioritise their baby's well-being above their own in all choice and decision-making throughout the maternity period.

> I mean I was upset because things weren't going to plan and I don't like that and then I just thought he's got to come out and that's the main thing and he's gonna be alright and that's the most important thing just get on with it. [Jane_4_1]

Despite the disempowerment that some women clearly experienced, a good outcome particularly when women are labelled as **abnormal pregnant women** and situated as **maternity patients** acknowledges the *experts* as playing a heroic role.

> I was quite frightened at that time about Josh I mean and my baby was paramount, more important than me. I happily relinquished that responsibility; they were brilliant all the midwives were great and the doctor. [Mary_4_1]

Experts, despite claims to support choice in pregnancy, retain control over when choice is appropriate for women and hold the power to remove choice. Women through their **good mother** identity prioritise their babies and relegate their own personal desires, which consequently reinforces the role of *experts* in retaining control over women's maternity care and choice.

CHOICE AND SATISFACTION

Choice that is offered in early pregnancy has been illuminated as complex and certainly not the simple concept that is presented to women. *Consumerist and feminist discourses* play roles in constructing women as desiring the right to make choices about the type of birth experience they want. Many women, however, make choices with no real knowledge of what is ahead in pregnancy or labour, and choices made based on the type of experience desired, for example *commodified notions of childbirth*, may not be fulfilled. When events mirror the choices they have made, women are generally more satisfied as seen in Mary and Polly's account below. Indeed women's narratives mirror their rationale for choosing a certain type of care and site of delivery, and demonstrate they made the responsible choices of a **good mother**.

> No I was happy really with everything, although my GP would want to see me next time apparently he likes to see his pregnant ladies but I didn't know, I was really happy with the midwives they're more confident anyway and whenever they were concerned they referred me. I still would have made the choice to deliver at the main unit regardless of my blood pressure I felt happier having that safety net, I mean I was happy with the midwives but then the doctors were around just in case. [Mary_4_1]

> [W]ith regard to the labour I was happy all the way through and happy with the midwife although I liked the reassurance of the doctor. [Polly_4_1]

Helen, following a third normal delivery despite having been labelled as an **abnormal pregnant women**, now claims she feels empowered to challenge the system. By denying *expert* labelling three times and proving herself a **normal pregnant woman** she feels authorised to demand the type of delivery that she feels would be best for her, her baby and her existing family. She reiterates here the role of the *GP gatekeeper* as a barrier to choice. Her earlier narratives, however, demonstrate that previous normal deliveries did not facilitate her ability to be assertive, constrained by notions of responsibility and fears of being labelled as a **bad mother**. This illustrates how barriers to choice are multifaceted and illuminates some of the difficulties this presents in offering real choice.

> I'd want a home birth this time, next time, I mean, if I had another one, I would elect for home birth but I wasn't given that choice, I was basically told that if I made that choice he wouldn't be my GP. [I: Would you act differently another time?] Yeah I would I'd put my foot down and demand a home birth. If you're not going to be my GP fine, I'll find another one that will . . . I mean I've had three, I've had no complications, they've all been early but no complications. [Helen_4_1]

Jane's narrative is an example of those women who suffered from unfulfilled choice. Her story exemplifies how the concept of choice can be unrealistic.

> I don't think we realised how big a thing it was and nobody can say this will happen and that will happen and that's the worst thing you just don't know what's gonna happen to you, you can have all the birth plans in the world but potentially it can still go wrong. [Jane_4_1]

The result of unfulfilled choice for Jane is a sense of failure to achieve the natural birth that had been offered by options for care. This *idealised notion of birth* that natural is better generates a **failed woman** identity in women who feel they missed an experience that is fundamental to their womanhood.

> I would still choose to have a natural one at the birth centre I'd still like to experience that and I feel a bit robbed in a way that I haven't experienced it. [Jane_4_1]

Mary equally suggests that natural creates a greater sense of satisfaction and achievement.

> [Y]ou know given the choice I would have wanted a natural, you've got to try. [Mary_4_1]

Choice is presented to women as a simple consumerist decision that asks them to consider the lead carer during pregnancy and birth environment, linked to the type of maternity experience to which they aspire. These women's narratives have consistently shown, however, that choice and decision-making in pregnancy is much more intricate. What seems significant here is in offering choice, the failure or refusal to fulfil that promise has clear ramifications which may have more negative repercussions than never offering choice at all.

WHAT ABOUT POSTNATAL CHOICE?

Women's accounts throughout have demonstrated the role of *societal depictions of motherhood* and the standards that women feel compelled to achieve in order to depict themselves as **good mothers**. Many women perceived postnatal input as significant in facilitating their **good mother** status. Postnatal care is the one aspect of maternity care in which women, until recently, have been offered no real choice. Care is provided by the midwife for a maximum of 28 days following birth and often removed earlier based on the midwife's judgement of the mother's needs.[1] However, the contemporary reality is that postnatal visiting at home has been cut back to the minimum and new initiatives such as postnatal clinics have come into being. The puerperium involves the maternal recovery from labour as well as adaptation to the role of **a real mother**. Studies have heralded modern maternity care as highlighting the social and psychological aspects of care, reducing emphasis on physical care in the postnatal period.[2] In contrast to the constructions of women's health in pregnancy and during birth, it is assumed that postnatal recovery is more rapid and requires much less in the way of care.[3] Mary narrates how such an approach left her feeling uncared for, unsure of what was expected of her and unsupported in her attempts to be a **good mother** and care for her baby following surgery.

> [T]he community midwives were great but the care on the postnatal ward was a bit inconsistent, it depended who was on really. I mean they were obviously really busy but sometimes I was just left on my own some shifts, I was okay but I did think gosh if I was on any other ward I wouldn't be doing so much after abdominal surgery. I mean the first day I got up and bathed him and everything, I felt great but I did suffer that night I was really stiff and in a lot of pain, but no-one told me how much to do. The midwife that night was really nice, she gave me an injection and it was fabulous but then I asked for one the next night and the midwife was horrified 'oh no you don't need an injection' and she gave me two tablets instead, she made me feel like a wimp really, I felt awful for asking. [Mary_4_1]

Polly goes further and implicates the postnatal staff as detrimental to her **good mother** status through their failure to support her to breastfeed.

> The only thing I would do differently was on the postnatal side . . . Next time I'd just really like to crack the breastfeeding and you don't get the one to one on the postnatal . . . I felt that if I rung the bell I was a burden and that everything you had to do for your baby was up to you and I think if I'd had more time in

> that first 48 hours trying to resolve the feeding issue that I wouldn't have had the problems when I got home. [Polly_4_1]

Sophie narrates an almost complete absence of care. Her account here suggests that midwives use their expertise to make judgements about who is the most deserving of their support, which does not involve any consultation with the mothers about their personal needs for care and support.

> I was put in a four-bedder completely on my own but I felt a bit in the middle of nowhere and I only buzzed once and they came but I never saw them again maybe they think it's because it's not your first that you can just get on with it. [Sophie_4_1]

All the above accounts narrate of an *absent expert*, who fails to support the women in their own recovery and return to **non-pregnant woman**. Kate describes how postnatal care gave no consideration to her personal needs and afforded her no choice in decision-making .

> I didn't like it there [the postnatal ward], the only down thing was when you want to go I got told in the morning I could go home but I didn't get to go until later on in the day so I'd rather they didn't say anything to you at all. [Kate_4_1]

Helen narrates a different story of satisfaction with the postnatal care. Her increased input, however, was based on a clear clinical need for *expert* involvement and care.

> Yeah I wasn't really in long enough to find out but they were alright, real nice and that and the after care was alright as well. The midwives who came to see me at home were real nice . . . she (health visitor) always pops in cos she knows I was postnatal (depressed) so she pops in about once a fortnight to make sure that I'm still here, to make sure I haven't done anything daft, yeah she's real nice. So my postnatal care has been better than before she was born. [Helen_4_1]

Sally in contrast felt that the midwife, through *expert* judgement, withdrew postnatal care at a time when she still felt the need for support. Sally given a choice would have preferred continued input.

> You had all this midwife coming round and people coming round then it all stops and leaves a big gap . . . everything just seemed to stop. [Sally_4_1]

Women's narratives suggest that postnatal input both in the hospital and in the community plays a key role in women's early adjustment to **a real mother** identity. Beyond that they believe it is fundamental in helping them to achieve a **good mother** identity. Postnatal care presents no real choice in a maternity culture, where choice, although often elusive, is being actively promoted. Women receive significant input during both the antenatal period and labour, yet at a point where support is perceived by them as equally if not more important and as integral to their **good mother** identities, skills and self-confidence, women feel let down and disappointed.

MATERNITY EXPERIENCE, CHOICE AND POSTNATAL DEPRESSION

Choice promotes a relationship with increased control, which in turn is assumed to lead to improved quality of experience and care, and perceived to lead to positive psychological health. Such an assumed framework makes this aspect worthy of further exploration. Four of the women, Helen, Sally, Jane and Sophie, suffered from significant but differing levels of emotional distress post-delivery. Helen and Sally were both clinically diagnosed with postnatal depression and their narratives will be explored in depth in order to further explicate the findings from the quantitative study. What became apparent in trying to provide some interpretation of these experiences is the contrast between the women's stories when relating their experiences but also the evident similarities. What is also marked is the need to consider women's pregnancy, birth and postnatal experience as a whole, and the complex interplay of women's individual physical, social and personal biographic realities.

Helen's story has featured throughout this chapter. Her maternity narrative to date tells of an unwanted pregnancy, plagued by physical health difficulties. Categorised and reinforced throughout her pregnancy by *experts* as an **abnormal pregnant woman**, she felt unfairly labelled and devoid of a real choice. Her wishes for a birth-centre delivery remained unfulfilled, premature labour situated her as a **maternity patient** and although her labour was clinically straightforward, it is generally described in negative terms. Experiences throughout pregnancy challenged her **good mother** identity and promoted her fears of being a **bad mother**. In the early postnatal period Helen's baby daughter became ill and was hospitalised, leaving Helen with a dominant **bad mother** identity infused with feelings of guilt and failure. Her late postnatal account tells a story of complete exhaustion and is consistent with the findings of Graham cited by Gatrell who described women as feeling a responsibility to 'keep going', leading them to try and ignore fatigue, amongst other physical symptoms.[4] Her narrative epitomises this claim but also demonstrates how the 'keeping going' is through a continued need to promote a **good mother** identity. Here the pressure of being a **good mother** to her new baby, conflicts with her need to be a **good mother** to her other children and to continue to effectively perform her perceived domestic labour role.

> [T]he first 4 months she was an absolute nightmare. She was asleep all day and awake all night. She would literally come to life at 10 p.m. and not go back to sleep until 6 a.m. No matter what you did to keep her awake during the day nothing worked . . . [I: How did you manage?] With great difficulty! I just never got any sleep at all . . . during the day I'd go to bed as soon as she went up in the morning and then the housework was piling up so I was doing the housework at like 2 a.m. and 3 a.m., ironing, washing and cleaning to get it done but she was 17 weeks before she slept through. She was asleep during the day no bother but night time . . . even during the day I wasn't getting much rest either, I mean she'd go over at 6 a.m. and then the other two were getting up . . . Knackered! I felt really, I didn't know what day of the week it was. [Helen_4_1]

Helen's feelings of inadequacy build on early guilt that she had been a **bad mother** not instinctively noticing an early postnatal problem, which resulted in her baby being hospitalised. This comment that 'she's gonna be one of these babies' acknowledges her attempts to provide an alternative explanation for her baby's behaviour, which she as a **good mother** should have recognised as abnormal. Explanation for this normalising of her baby's behaviour, however, could feasibly be grounded in Helen's late-pregnancy narrative. In late pregnancy we saw Helen begin to determine her baby's characteristics, by using the adjective 'awkward'. This labelling of her baby continues into the postnatal period and results in a failure to recognise a problem, which despite seeking *expert* advice, Helen takes complete responsibility for.

> I blame myself in a way because I think why didn't I pick up on it? I mean she was born the Tuesday and I had a real bad night with her the Tuesday night, not really feeding properly just about 5 minutes, she wasn't really feeding properly and she was crying all night, and I just thought a new baby she's gonna be one of these babies and then Wednesday night she was a bit better but a bit the same and Thursday she wasn't very well and I spoke to the midwife and the midwife said she's probably got jaundice but I did sort of feel it was my fault I should've taken her on the Wednesday and said I think there's something the matter with her, I just ignored it really. [Helen_4_1]

Sally's maternity profile is entirely different to Helen's. Her initial thoughts about her pregnancy were somewhat ambivalent, however, her pregnancy and birth experience were generally good and she was satisfied with the choices she made for care. Interpretation of her postnatal depression seems apparent in her articulation of the whole experience of **a real mother** as a new social role completely overwhelming and traumatic. Her narrative is infused with feelings of vulnerability, loneliness and isolation, which in addition highlight the failure of postnatal aftercare to adequately assess her psychological health needs and necessary input in the postnatal period

> I just felt really miserable, everything in my life had changed completely it was just me and her, I couldn't go anywhere or do anything I just felt also I missed people because I'd always worked with people and I just felt really isolated, I felt I needed people around me but it was like a chicken and egg because the minute they disappeared I just sit down and start crying really really crying. [Sally_4_1]

Sophie had a good pregnancy but as shown previously a negative birth experience, created by the feeling of loss of choice and control during pregnancy. Her own account does not make a direct link between her experiences and her subsequent emotional response, nor does she describe herself as depressed, but she does articulate a state of emotional vulnerability that is out of character.

> I would have days where I'd just have outbursts of tears and then I'd take it out on Karl and then I'd be crying in bed which just wasn't me you know I'd never been like that before. [Sophie_4_1]

Interestingly Jane, who in the early postnatal period was very emotionally distressed and tearful about the lack of control and loss of choice she experienced in labour, is in the late postnatal period much more pragmatic. The enduring emotional impact of her experience is evident in her decision not to have more children, yet her narrative does not display the emotional vulnerability visible in Sophie's account.

> Oh yeah I'm alright about it now, as you can see I'm not in tears, I've got over that . . . I'm over it now, it's still upsetting and I'm still not planning another one . . . we don't dwell on it but if it's brought up its still distressing. [Jane_4_1]

The guilt inherent in Helen's previous account is also evident in Sally's narrative below, although revealed in a different context. Here *cultural standards of bonding,* which influenced women during pregnancy, feature strongly in positioning Sally as a **bad mother**. She articulates feelings of failure, exacerbated by the reaction of others around her, hence sending her further down the spiral of emotional distress.

> I think the worst bit was that I felt I wasn't bonding with her and then I started to get upset about that because it was another stress because everybody bonds, I didn't feel I wanted to play with her or do things with her, my Mum said one day I was lucky to be able to spend time with her and I said 'I'm not lucky' and she was really upset . . . I just felt so low and isolated and I thought nobody understood and I also felt like I was the only one and I thought as a mother this shouldn't be happening you should be bonding with your baby. [Sally_3_1]

Pressure from significant others also featured significantly in Helen's narrative. Here, she refers to pressure exerted by her partner. Her account echoes the traditional construct of the woman as **the domestic labourer**,[4] despite the demands of new motherhood and the specific difficulties encountered by Helen following the birth of her daughter. This confounds her feelings of failure and results in worryingly irrational and extreme thoughts.

> Yeah, yeah, I would have tried anything including jumping off the . . . bridge. I would have tried anything and he was getting on my back when he came back from work on a weekend saying the house was a tip, can't you do no bloody cleaning these days. [Helen_4_1]

As discussed by other authors the *gendered discourse* that traditionally depicts women as responsible for childcare and domestic tasks was evident.[4] Sophie reflects Helen's positioning of her as **the domestic labourer** by her husband:

> [H]e's got it easy and sometimes he'll say you don't do any tidying up and I think god if that's all you've got to worry . . . [Sophie_4_1]

The **domestic labourer** identity was particularly evident in the narratives of women suffering emotional distress post-delivery. This fostered resentment towards their partners, which was expressed, but the perceived inequity, although questioned, did not appear to be fundamentally addressed with their partners. It is possible that this failure to challenge is a consequence of their emotionally vulnerable state.

> I was thinking I've got three kids, nobody to help me, he's never at home to help me, he's only home at a weekend, she's like she was, I wasn't getting any sleep,

so . . . [I: Did you feel quite resentful towards your husband then?] To start with yeah, even when he came home on a weekend, he wouldn't do anything on a weekend he works all week and doesn't see why he should have the kids on a weekend . . . he doesn't see why he should have to get up and sort her in the night . . . I mean it wouldn't have hurt him to get up, you know . . . while I went to bed for 12 hours but he wouldn't do it. [I: Did he not realise how difficult it was for you?] Well he did but, he just classes it as he works all week and I don't do anything so . . . he works all week so his weekends are his time for relaxing and unwinding. [Helen_4_1]

Partners as in the early postnatal period are cited as unprepared for and insensitive to the adjustment in social identity that goes with motherhood, compounding the emotional distress women experienced. Sally narrates how once again the *institution and ideologies of motherhood* place demands and expectations on women that are beyond those associated with fatherhood. This account reports a continuation of the lack of being cared for, that many women articulated in the early postnatal period.

I felt that John wanted this baby but it was me stuck with her and doing everything, his life hadn't changed and mine had changed so dramatically and I just felt so low and isolated and I thought nobody understood and I also felt like I was the only one and I thought as a mother this shouldn't be happening to you. I sometimes found him not as supportive as he could have been, I found my Mum and Dad supportive . . . I needed looking after and he couldn't do that and because I had my Mum and Dad he didn't feel obliged even now he doesn't understand . . . I really don't think men can understand it and I think they could do with education a bit more. [Sally_4_1]

Jane, however, recognises that it is her compliance with the social constraints of *gendered parenting discourses* in identifying herself as a **good mother** that dictated her postnatal emotional adjustment, rather than a failure on her husband's part to meet the expectations of his role as *a father*.

I think the smallest things like if Paul was late home from work I'd just create and I can't really explain why I was like that . . . his life hadn't changed at all he could still go climbing and play football and I couldn't go out because I had to feed Luke and I felt awful I shouldn't feel like that but I did start to resent it . . . it was me feeling guilty and even asking Paul to have him I was bigging it up if you like that I shouldn't want to leave him. [Jane _4_1]

Partners exerted other additional pressures, which challenged women's tentative **good mother** identities, as in Sally's account. She feels threatened by her husband's apparent ease and ability to bond with their daughter, and the relationship that is evolving between the two.

> I always feel like every now and again I have to step back he'll walk through the door and she's laughing I am bonding with her now definitely but she doesn't laugh as much with me and I have to take a step back and think I'm not such a bad mother I care for her and feed her and just because I don't make her laugh 24 hours a day doesn't make me a bad mother and that was another thing I was beating myself up over. [Sally_4_1]

The guilt that infuses these narratives is exacerbated by feelings that women have no right to feel miserable or unable to cope and that they should be grateful for a healthy baby, particularly when there is no identified tangible reason for depression, as in Sophie's case.

> [J]ust crying because I felt miserable but there wasn't really a particular problem, people would think what's your problem with Billy he's such an easy baby but there was just lots of things. [Sophie_4_1]

> You get this little person and your world turns upside down and I just couldn't get over how I was an intelligent person with a good job and yet I couldn't cope . . . I had more company than I'd ever had yet I felt so lonely. [Sally_4_1]

All women expressed feelings of loneliness and isolation.

> I think I just needed adult conversation more than anything, I think that's what I really needed. I'd had the kids all week and he's home on a weekend and I've still got the kids, if I was going anywhere it was like take all the kids with you and I just didn't get any adult conversation. [Helen_4_1]

> I just felt really miserable, everything in my life had changed completely it was just me and her, I couldn't go anywhere or do anything I just felt also I missed people because I'd always worked with people and I just felt really isolated. [Sally_4_1]

Work is mentioned by Sally above and clearly articulated by Sophie as a way of regaining the 'personal identity', the **me** they perceive they have lost following the *birth of the baby*.

> I do feel a bit lonely and think there must be more, I do think god it will be nice to get back to work just to be around adult people. I do see my friends but just to do something different. [Sophie_4_1]

Jane's narrative demonstrates how returning to work was key in regaining her **me** identity and perhaps affords some explanation of why her emotional distress despite a traumatic delivery was less enduring.

> I needed adult conversation I mean even though I was seeing adults everyday all the conversations revolved around Luke and its nice to go to work I knew I had to get back to work even now months on I am getting out and Paul is very good but . . . I'm only just starting to get my own life back. [Jane_4_1]

It is significant that Helen, Sally and Sophie narrate the difficulty of openly acknowledging mental health problems and the stigma associated with antidepressants.

> I didn't tell my husband I was on them though, he is one of these that doesn't believe in things like that he thinks it's just a cop out of saying that you can't cope. [Helen_4_1]

> [C]lose people said go to the doctors but I didn't want to go down that line because once you start on tablets that I can't get off and then going back to work on antidepressants won't do me any good but its gone full circle and me and Karl have been talking more. [Sophie_4_1]

Sally articulates a desire to avoid been labelled as 'postnatally depressed'.

> It took me a while to go to the doctors because I really didn't want to go down that route but I did because I just needed to get on with my life. [Sally_4_1]

Helen narrates how behaviour can become extreme in the face of postnatal depression and how this behaviour finally revealed the severity of the situation.

> I think the final straw for me was before I went to the doctors, he came in at tea time and said I want my tea on the table at 5 o'clock and he sat down . . . at the

table so I did put his dinner on the table, meat, peas, carrots, gravy all on the table and he said what's this, and I said you never said you wanted a plate, you wanted your dinner on the table so there it is on the table and the kids were sat there howling with laughter. And he said I think you should see a doctor and that was the final straw cos I thought maybe I have gone a bit over the top . . . I locked myself in the bathroom and cried my eyes out, I was in floods of tears and I wouldn't open the door for about half an hour. [Helen_4_1]

Both Helen and Sally's accounts tell of a frightening reality that made it imperative to seek some help. Although previous work has suggested that GPs often fail to take women's depression seriously,[5] both Helen and Sally found support from their GPs

I mean it had got to the stage where I was screaming blue murder, I could've killed the kids I really could've. It got to the stage where all they'd do is walk past and I'd just scream at them, throwing pots and smashing them, and I'd walk into town and burst into tears in the middle of Woolies, I just felt absolutely awful. And I just went to the doctors and told him how I felt and he put me on the tablets. [Helen_4_1]

I ended up living at my Mum's for 3 months, I got worse as the weeks went on . . . but then they were going away and I needed to be able to cope on my own and so I went to see the doctor and he put me on some tablets basically and they've been brilliant I'm still on them now. [Sally_4_1]

Despite the support experienced from their GPs neither Helen nor Sally were offered any alternatives to medication. Both, interestingly, have gone on to build their own informal support networks, which seem to address the isolation and loneliness aspects of suffering postnatal depression.

[W]e get together every week, every Tuesday and there's a woman whose husband works offshore so she understands and I feel its not just me because we talk about babies, we talk about other things but we talk about how we feel as well so its just good support. [Sally_4_1]

I have coffee mornings across the road when the kids are at school. [I: Is that a friendship you've built up since you've had her?] No we've always been friends, but since I've had her obviously I couldn't really do it because she was always asleep during the day, she was always in bed so it's only in the last few months that I've been able to start going across. [Helen_4_1]

Women with postnatal depression remain plagued by *ideologies of motherhood, gendered parenting discourses* and *traditional notions of domestic women*, positioning themselves as **bad mothers** during their period of depression, out of control and unable to function effectively in their role as **a real mother**.

> I felt like I'd jumped out of an aeroplane and the parachute was failing, I couldn't get control of anything, the house, the kids, the dog, I just couldn't shake it off and I was thinking why am I getting out of bed this morning, I just didn't want to get up, didn't want to go out. [Helen_4_1]

> I feel guilty that for the first few months she was shunted around just to be with people and I didn't interact with her and I felt guilty and now I feel better I've decided to take the year off to make up that lost time with her. [Sally_4_1]

The context of the emotional distress articulated by these women was very different and evolved out of a milieu of individual antenatal, intranatal and postnatal events, circumstances and adjustment following delivery. The women themselves did not directly attribute their psychological distress post-delivery to any pregnancy or labour events or to unfulfilled choices, they saw their distress merely in the context of postnatal events. Failure to fulfil choice whilst seeming to impact on some women's emotional maternity experience is only one of the many negative factors experienced by these women and cannot, in these narratives, be attributed the status of a single causative factor. The guilt, sense of failure, loneliness, isolation, loss of control, inability to cope, loss of personal identity, stigma and lack of support that is inherent in the experience of postnatal depression displayed in these women's narratives is both frightening and distressing. The continued perfusion of many idealised societal discourses position these women as **bad mothers**, at a time when they lack the emotional resources to restore their **good mother** identities; as they are equally struggling to cope with the physical recovery of pregnancy and permanent tiredness, compounding the downward spiral of psychological distress. Their accounts clearly support an individual, multidimensional, psychosocial model of postnatal depression. Unless necessity forced them to seek help, there was no accessible postnatal aftercare other than routine care. This is withdrawn, based on *expert* judgement rather than through an interactive and negotiated discussion with the woman. Particularly for this small yet extremely vulnerable group of women, this appears to be a serious omission in the choice debate.

SUMMARY

These late postnatal reflections highlight the embedded nature of experts and expertise within women's labour experiences, reinforcing the early postnatal suggestion that the consumerist choice discourse in maternity has not been accompanied by a fundamental shift in power away from experts to women. Expert knowing maps onto women's aspirations to be **good mothers** and constrains their ability to exercise their rights, maintain control and make choices. Women throughout their maternity experience have demonstrated that they sit within a complex matrix of influences and discourses. Within this multifaceted environment for many women, choice is often an elusive or unfulfilled concept, the ramifications of which clearly merit further consideration. The choice discourse furthermore fails women in the postnatal period. In contrast to the expertise that assails them in pregnancy and labour, the postnatal period is depicted as a time of minimal support that is often withdrawn without any consultation with the woman herself. For those women who suffered postnatal emotional distress their narratives depict a complex psychosocial experience in which societal discourses position them as **bad mothers**, and the promotion of themselves as **good mothers** becomes increasingly difficult.

REFERENCES

1 Silverton L. *The Art and Science of Midwifery*. Hemel Hempstead: Prentice Hall; 1993.
2 Ball JA. Mothers need nurturing too. *Nursing Times*. 1988; 84(27): 29–31.
3 Woollett A, Marshall H. Motherhood and mothering. In: Ussher JM, editor. *Women's Health: contemporary international health perspectives*. Leicester: The British Psychological Society; 2000.
4 Gatrell C. *Hard Labour: the sociology of parenthood*. Maidenhead: Open University Press; 2005.
5 Kitzinger S. *Ourselves as Mothers*. London: Doubleday; 1992.

CHAPTER 9

Choice, control and contemporary childbirth

It has been demonstrated through women's subjective accounts that choice is a far more complex phenomenon than both policy-makers and consumerist discourse suggest and would have women believe. Maternity choice is presented as a simple concept that involves women making decisions based on information given in order to facilitate a desired pregnancy and birth experience, increase personal control and promote satisfaction resulting in subsequent emotional well-being. Interpretation of the quantitative findings of this study[1] demonstrated that offering choice of carer or place of birth per se fails to impact on positive psychological outcomes and that no one care option confers any significant psychological benefit. It is apparent, that such simplicity is not reflected in women's experiences. For women making maternity choices, there are inherent tensions. Desires are themselves multifaceted; surreptitious influences affect women's actions and decisions; and choice also includes risk assessment and a rational thought process, which results in an ordering of preferences.

That changes in service delivery have occurred facilitated the very undertaking of this study. However, this leads to other fundamental questions, which are, firstly, whether this has led to a major rethinking of the way in which pregnancy and childbirth are now perceived, and, secondly, whether women have secured autonomy and veracity within the new maternity services. Choice is now a concept firmly embedded in the societal discourse that surrounds care during pregnancy and birth, and as such has become not only expected and desired by women, but also, as this study has shown, another normative requirement to which women need to conform. Indeed, the establishment of choice as another idealised norm, in opposition to the claim that choice increases satisfaction and emotional well-being, can be seen to create additional pressures for some women who feel that they must firstly not only prove themselves as normal, but maintain that normality in order to realise their idealised maternity experience through choice. For others, their choices are made on the premise that normality cannot be assured until after birth. For these women they can only consider themselves normal after birth when everything has gone to plan (if it has). This group of women consider pregnancy and birth as something potentially problematic and as such choose to deliver at a hospital unit to have a safety net. This inference is underpinned by the powerful nature of idealised normative representations of maternity that women construct themselves within and through, and which inherently make choice complex.

As this book has suggested from the start, women are not the homogeneous group that the choice discourse assumes. Health policy[2] and Maternity Matters[3] both acknowledge that social inequalities in income, housing and nutrition inherently restrict choice and access to services. Indeed it has been claimed that 'choice in maternity care is really a choice for the articulate middle classes' (p. 7).[4] The findings of this study, however, have revealed other more embedded, less explicit, constraints to choice that apply to a broader group of women. These implicit constraints exist in the form of the discourses, and influences construct normative and idealised identities that demand conformity from women and can be elucidated through women's pregnancy narratives.

For all the women interviewed, the part played by the fetus in situating them in a mothering role from almost the earliest point in their pregnancies was a consistent narrative. Pregnancy has long been acknowledged as a transition stage in women's lives.[5] Birth, however, has been traditionally recognised as the point at which mothering starts,[6] and few writers have acknowledged pregnancy as the beginning of mothering. What seems apparent for women is that the recognition of themselves as pregnant creates a vision of the fetus as a life they have created and thus a baby. Narratives show that from almost the earliest point in their pregnancies women begin to consider how having a baby will impact on their lives. They articulate worries about how they will cope with a new baby through the recognition that following a positive pregnancy test they are different to what they were before.

Conceptualising themselves as mothers to their fetuses, in this way, quickly invests them with an inherent personal responsibility and accountability analogous to that expected from mothers. The pressure to provide care to their fetuses that conforms to the standards of good mothering is apparent even within the first trimester of pregnancy. Whilst women clearly aspire to be a good mother and a responsible pregnant women, they wrestle with other identities, such as normal and abnormal pregnant woman, which remain predominantly defined through a medical model, where the woman is regarded as the vessel of containment for the fetus and at the mercy of unpredictable forces that might endanger the contents of the vessel.[7] Within this framework, birth remains conceptualised by women as unknown and unpredictable, and by some as inherently risky and potentially feared. Women's narratives present a complex picture where numerous circulating discourses and influences are absorbed, accepted or resisted to provide justification for the choices they make.

The dominant drive to adopt the characteristics intrinsic in good mothering and to meet the ideology of motherhood is a key influence in women's experiences from the earliest point. This identity causes women to represent themselves within constructed childbirth norms, demonstrate advocacy and make responsible choices that prioritise the well-being of their babies. This, as a consequence, renders personal desires for a pregnancy and birth experience, which inform a key premise of maternity choice, less important although not non-existent. Whilst women clearly have personal desires about type of birth experience and environment for birth and pain relief, needs are ranked and predominantly rationalised through a safety premise. Thus, birth choices involve no fundamental rejection of professional input, which is embedded in women's minds as the way to ensure a healthy birth outcome. Expert advice is sought, and recommendations for care are mostly listened to. Whilst these women are perceived to have made choices about their maternity care, they have often been presented with recommended care options rather than alternatives of care set out in the context of advantages and disadvantages, leaving the woman to make the decision. This is a key aspect of the maternity experience that clearly makes it difficult for women to have legitimate, meaningful and beneficial choice.

CHOICE AND CONTROL

Women in early pregnancy narratives do not dwell on labour; however, narratives in late pregnancy demonstrate that thoughts and fears about the impending labour become more prominent. Some late-pregnancy fears and worries reflect early pregnancy concerns about choice of site for delivery and women express concerns about not meeting the 'normal pregnant woman' standards that would facilitate their choice. Other worries articulated, however, are more concerned with expectations of the birth experience itself and conforming to depictions of a 'controlled labourer'. Maintaining control and coping in labour were central to women's labour expectation narratives, as they felt pressured to conform to the composed and calm depiction of a 'good mother' even in labour. Worries were generated by experienced labour discourses, which were predominantly 'horror stories' and were incompatible with women's desires to have a 'normal and natural' delivery. Additional fears about labour interventions and mode of delivery are also prominent within women's accounts, consistent with studies which found that late pregnancy was a time when worries increase[1] and that giving birth was one of the most widespread sources of extreme worry,[7,8] so in that sense could be considered unsurprising.

Lowe's suggestion that fear and apprehension regarding labour were associated with high levels of external control adds another interesting interpretive dimension to the issue of choice and control.[9] Fear and apprehension causes women to willingly cede control to experts and, indeed, they both expect and desire to do so, particularly in late pregnancy and labour. They do, however, express desires to control how and to whom the mantle is handed over and it seems that choices are partly made on that premise. This rationale remains entrenched in the powerful way that pregnancy, birth and postnatal recovery are both constructed and represented within society. Women are driven to make responsible choices to assert their 'good mother' status, but responsible choices in turn remain informed by a depiction of birth as hazardous and the domain of 'expert knowing'. Choice gives women an active role in their maternity experience, but also leaves them open to criticism of making the wrong choice, that is, one that might endanger their babies. Women fundamentally, whilst often having a desired ideal experience, see challenging expert knowing, particularly in the face of a pregnancy or labour problem, as a risk that they are generally unprepared to take. The inherently problematic image of childbirth and the consequent expert management is embedded in women's minds.

Whilst those women choosing the birth centre could be viewed as opting for a less medicalised approach to their delivery, in a less hospitalised environment, it remains nevertheless perceived as an environment of expertise. Midwifery-led care is envisioned by women as a route to a more normal and natural pregnancy and birth experience, within a safe framework of expertise. Midwives and doctors are consistently united under the heading of 'experts,' and expert intervention within the maternity arena remains fundamentally unchallenged by women. Midwives, whilst often associated with normality by women, in the face of 'deviation from the norm' retain 'expert knowing,' enabling them to identify women as 'abnormal pregnant women' and to situate them as 'maternity patients'. This increases the amount of control that they, as midwives, exercise over women and as such is likely to at least reduce or at worst remove completely women's choice and control over pregnancy events.

Further the identification, in women's accounts, of the midwife as the pregnancy 'expert' and the first point of call in the face of a problem in pregnancy potentially negates the suggestion that offering midwifery-led alternatives for care allows women to make choices that facilitate increased levels of personal control. Noteworthy, however, is the argument that women in pregnancy and childbirth actually make a conscious decision to hand over elements of personal control, whether to a midwife or a doctor.[10] Narrative accounts here also support the notion that whilst there is an increase in control by 'powerful others' across pregnancy and in labour, this may not be the detrimental decision that has previously been suggested. The women's accounts demonstrate that they make decisions about when they feel they wish to relinquish control. The women established that this can happen in pregnancy either for reassurance of normality or through a pregnancy related problem, where their need to be a 'good mother' and ensure the well-being of their baby supersedes the desire to maintain personal control. This willing surrender of control is also depicted in their reflections on labour, again, emerging for some women out of the actions of a 'good mother' or because of pain. These accounts seem to support the argument that external control is not always unwelcome to women. Women openly articulate that they look for guidance from the midwife. Further, many women have made care package choices based on the premise that as 'good mothers' they are prepared to relinquish control to the 'experts' at any point in their pregnancies to ensure the well-being of their babies.

Pain was another important factor associated with maintaining control in labour, and for some women choices for care was based on the availability of pain relief to facilitate a controlled labourer identity. External control again in this context was not unwelcome. This is reinforced by labour narratives in which 'experts' were praised when they facilitated women's requests for pain relief and castigated when they failed to do so, as the previous findings of Mander[11] and Green and Baston[10] have also suggested.

Apparent in the 'reflecting on labour' narratives, and probably relevant to pregnancy as well, is that it is not being located as a 'maternity patient' by the midwife per se that impacts on women's sense of control, but rather how that transfer to 'maternity patient' is handled. Although the language used by experts can be seen in women's accounts to be disempowering and detrimental to personal control, if camouflaged within a remit of caring, women do not articulate it as a problem or as feeling deprived of control. Some women who criticised their labour experience did narrate feeling uncared for. Overall, however, women's accounts in this study with regard to labour, whether they felt they had retained control or not, ultimately narrated positively about the 'experts' involved.

The expectation and desire for professional input in pregnancy is firmly embedded in women's minds, regardless of choices for care and is clearly reflected in the stories women tell. Indeed, women feel uncared for and let down when needs and expectations for professional input are unmet. Choice and control are linked in women's minds and women seem to believe that one facilitates the other. Involving women in choice and control aspects of their maternity experience has been part of the shift towards an acknowledgement of the psychology of childbirth. Choice, as highlighted in the introduction to this book, is a concept that aims to facilitate women's desires for the amount of control they wish to receive,[12] in recognition that negative perceptions of care and lack of control, particularly during labour and birth, can be detrimental to postnatal psychological well-being.[10] The women's stories told here add coherent extensions to those previous claims. Choice, more than facilitating women's desired birth experience, does appear to allow women to consider and make decisions about the professional input and type of control they desire or are prepared to accept, whatever their underpinning rationale. Control, however, takes many different guises and is about more than maintaining control over decision-making and maternity events, but is also conceptualised by women in other ways. Choices can also reflect desires, for example, to retain control in labour facilitated by pain relief. Choices for women may be less about maintaining personal control throughout pregnancy and birth or a rejection of expert knowing, as has been previously suggested, and more about options, as suggested by Renfrew and colleagues, that allow women to feel respected and treated as individuals in the manner in which they are handled by care givers [13]. Women are perhaps making decisions based on the type and amount of control they are willing to cede and to whom; therefore, they are largely satisfied because the levels and nature of control experienced are as expected. Choice should perhaps be discussed in terms of women's desires for control within their experience regardless of site for delivery, and not necessarily in terms of idealised birth experience.

DO MIDWIVES EQUAL CHOICE FOR WOMEN?

The powerful role played by the GP in facilitating or impeding women's choices at the earliest point based on perceived normality, has been previously acknowledged.[4] The recommendations of that report suggest this could be addressed by alternative models of care such as direct access to midwives, a service that has now commenced in many areas across the UK. It could be suggested that the development of these services and the subsequent change in the way many women now access maternity services, which now often excludes the GP, makes the narratives concerning the GP irrelevant. However, direct access schemes in the context of choice can learn many lessons from the stories that these women tell. Firstly, ensuring 'real choice' will require a culture change in women themselves; making choices and participating in decisions regarding maternity care remains an unusual and infrequent concept for women. Secondly, changes to practices and procedures will fail to address the problem if midwives themselves fail to accept the level of control they are perceived by women to hold or acknowledge that their professional attitudes are also culpable in restricting women's choices at the earliest point. As already suggested, midwives are linked by women to normal and natural childbirth, but paradoxically they are also clinical experts who, like the GP, can act as the mouthpiece of the medical model. As others have previously found and as has been referred to in earlier chapters, changing systems and places of birth does not inherently provide the answer to this paradox. Findings from this study appear to indicate that midwifery-led care is not as inevitably women-centred as advocates would suggest and does not automatically lead to increased personal control for women, which is also congruent with the findings of several other authors presented in the earlier chapters of this book. The direct access to midwives services currently being implemented across the UK should not automatically be assumed to offer greater access to 'real choice' for women. All care providers, including midwives, need to be aware of how they reinforce dominant childbirth norms and the influence they assert over women's choices. So long as doctors and midwives as experts continue to devalue and dismiss women's 'personal knowing' and assert themselves as experts, then the childbearing women's right to choice regarding their own personal care, is liable to be limited.

'SO HAVE I GOT A CHOICE?'

The hegemony of expertise, monitoring and surveillance in pregnancy and childbirth that occurs regardless of the type of care, undoubtedly facilitates the early recognition of abnormality. The ability to quickly identify and treat serious conditions or complications of pregnancy can claim success in reducing maternal and fetal mortality and morbidity. However, within a choice framework it creates difficulties for some women. Choice offered, within a framework of monitoring and potential abnormality, allows experts to rescind choice at any point during the pregnancy and birth experience.

Women's accounts indeed suggest that, for some, choice remains almost a luxury and a privilege rather than a right. Whilst the foundation of women's choices is so multifaceted and complex, choices made in early pregnancy with no knowledge of how the pregnancy will progress create a risk of unfulfilled choice. The ramifications of unfulfilled choice seem dependant on women's underpinning rationale for choice. A 'realistic vision' of choice as constrained by normality, and recognition that choice might be removed by experts under the premise of maternal of more importantly fetal wellbeing, appears to have less personal emotional consequences for women if and when choice is removed. However, there are also apparent emotional repercussions of unfulfilled choices.

For example, the tensions inherent between women's idealised notions of birth as normal and natural, and medicalised interventionalist approaches can generate more damaging emotional consequences than if choice was never offered. This can be exacerbated by the language that is used at the time when choice is being removed. The implications of promoting birth as fundamentally normal and natural whilst not being critiqued, as such, must recognise its impact on those women who fail to achieve a normal or natural pregnancy or birth. Choices to deliver under midwifery led care to provide access to pain relief and/ or feelings of safety should not be dismissed as less valid and choice discourses must acknowledge the legacy of the medical model within women's decision-making in pregnancy. The problem of unfulfilled choice and its potential negative consequences could be further addressed by providing women with information but not asking them to make a choice about site for delivery in early pregnancy. Choices should be made in light of pregnancy progress and events, and at a much later stage in pregnancy when choice can possibly be offered realistically to women.

The complexity of choice illuminated by the women's accounts in this study, suggests that theories of choice in maternity must be supported by empirical evidence, accrued from within sensitive research designs, with the ability to detect individual as well as the collective consequences of unfulfilled choice. Choice should be part of maternity care but this does demand that care providers are able to present a realistic and honest depiction of what choice means. Expectations of care and site of delivery need to be realistic within the present climate and not idealised. Consumerist discourse is currently misleading; choice is not currently 'a right' for all women and needs to be candidly acknowledged. Choice if rescinded should be done so with full understanding, cooperation and consent from the woman. Further, this requires a consideration of the language care givers use to deprive women of choice, which potentially affords the blame for unfulfilled choice to the woman herself. The potentially negative emotional consequences of unfulfilled choice should be understood, acknowledged and monitored by maternity care providers. Care providers should be openly accountable to women for limited or unfulfilled choice. In addition, valuable insight could be provided by future research, which considers the psychological outcomes and experiences of women openly excluded from choice due to medical or obstetric reasons.

Pregnant women regardless of their choices for care are bound by the psychological consequences of maternity discourses and influences, whether negative or positive. They are restricted by the limited images and descriptions of childbirth and motherhood to which they have access; by the attitudes and language of the health professionals who look after them, the continuation of maternity

he thing that 'good mothers' do. Midwives, paradoxically, however,
women as necessary and instrumental in achieving confidence and
e in caring for their babies. Hence midwives set the standards of good
but, due to lack of resource and the current system of service provi-
simultaneously provide insufficient care and support and position
'bad mothers'.

care reduces self worth by threatening the 'good mother' identity
dering feelings of failure and guilt. Potential explanations for the
ies between expectation and receipt of care can be proffered by the
naturalness of mothering, the focus of maternity care on the well-
safe delivery of the baby and the subsequent withdrawal of medical
llowing that outcome as well as the often inadequate resourcing of
services.

ults of this study have shown how personal and complex women's
t to motherhood is after birth. This highlights the need to focus atten-
e individuality of women's experiences, particularly important when
r is emotionally vulnerable due to factors or events over which she has
. The skills and tools to recognise emotional vulnerability across the
spectrum alongside providing negotiated levels of individual care in
tal period would seem to be the key to identifying potential postna-
logical distress. Psychological distress, however, is undeniably about
en themselves experience their pregnancies, relationships and indi-
nts over the whole maternity period. Further, the way in which care
d by midwives during the postnatal period has a clear and potentially
effect on women's emotional health. The failure to extend the con-
model into the postnatal period appears to be a failure of the system to
l its promise of choice and secondly an omission with consequences
uivocally requires attention.

RY

have the potential to make a significant difference to a woman's expe-
childbirth regardless of her choices for care. This is likely to operate at
erent levels, from the expert judgements that are made, the language
ed, how normality is presented, perceived and reinforced, how emo-
lnerability is recognised, understood and managed, to what extent
el they are being cared for and cared about, supported, and able to
isions affecting their care. Therefore, what an effective model of choice
s a greater understanding, acknowledgement and respect of the com-
how women understand and engage with not only their pregnancy,

care as a domain of expertise and the language to which women themselves
have access in order to express their emotional status.

EMOTIONAL STATUS AND CHOICE

Pregnancy is an acknowledged time of emotional lability for women, which
endures into the postnatal period. Choice, although not unimportant to women,
rather than facilitating desired experience often rather facilitates the necessity to
conform to desired idealised identities. It is the failure to meet these identities
that appears to mediate emotional distress and enduring psychological consequences rather than failures to fulfil a desired birth experience. This proffers a
further explanation for the lack of effect that choice of care as a single variable
has made to date with regard to psychological outcomes.[1,13] Emotional distress
when it does occur is individualised, disparate and emerges from a multifaceted
psychosocial matrix.

It seems imperative for the context of women's psychological health to
be understood from a perspective that takes account of their entire maternity
experience. The consumerist choice debate reinforced by policy, and academic
and popular literature depicts choice in maternity care as increasing satisfaction with pregnancy and birth experiences, and thus directly contributing to
emotional well-being.[14] For women who maintain normality and do not suffer
any challenges to their desired birth experience, it seems that this may well be
true. However, what is significant within women's subjective accounts is how
offering choice can conversely render other women disempowered, guilty, angry
and distressed. Women from the earliest point of contact are scrutinised under
a defined framework of normality. Those who expect, yet fail to meet the normality criteria at any point in their pregnancies are labelled as abnormal and
denied choice or charged with a remit of proving their normality before their
choices can be fulfilled.

Unfulfilled choice, whilst seemingly, for some women, playing a contributory role to subsequent psychological sequelae, cannot be given the standing of
a single causative factor. Women throughout their pregnancy strive to promote
themselves as 'good mothers', act responsibly and make appropriate decisions.
Many other discourses, influences and events serve to reinforce their status as
'good or bad mothers' throughout pregnancy. Women who maintain only a
tenuous grasp of their 'good mother' identity are rendered emotionally vulnerable as pregnancy progresses. It seems apparent that those women who leave
pregnancy emotionally vulnerable enter the postnatal period in the same state,
regardless of delivery events. Postnatal events build on this level of emotional
vulnerability, which appears to manifest in perceived failures to adequately fulfil

'good mother', 'gendered parenting' and 'domestic labourer' roles, perpetuating the descent into significant psychological distress.

For some women the location of emotional vulnerability is less apparent in their antenatal narratives, yet implicit in their postnatal accounts is a similar state of emotional vulnerability. This emerges from accounts of disappointing delivery experiences that did not meet with expectations and/or the overwhelming nature of being a 'real mother' characterised by loneliness, isolation and resentment. Many of these postnatal accounts are infused with some articulated loss of personal identity, as women feel constrained and pressured, in the postnatal period, by 'gendered parenting' and domestic labour roles. Resentment is articulated through narratives that compare female to male parenting roles. Whilst some women narrate an emotional vulnerability in the early postnatal period often as a result of individualised experiences, this emotional vulnerability does not manifest in enduring postnatal depression, suggesting that some women are equipped with better personal resources and are more empowered or enabled to restore personal identity than others. The differences among those women who narrated emotional distress and did not feel pushed to seek help and those who did, appears to be located in feelings of failure and inability to function rather than feelings of low mood. Those women pushed to seek help did so out of their perception of themselves as 'bad mothers' and an apparent inability to adequately fulfil idealised roles.

These accounts clearly illuminate a multifaceted image of postnatal depression. The privileged insight into postnatal depression that emerges from women's narratives appears to enable the conclusions that whilst women's accounts depict an individualised biography, they are underpinned by perceived failures to meet the idealised cultural and societal depictions that surround pregnancy and childbirth. There is no one consistent causative factor that characterises the experience of postnatal distress. The level of postnatal distress is perhaps mediated by personal resources, but is more clearly located in women's abilities to perform and perceive themselves as 'good mothers'. Hence, care givers need to be aware of the role they can play in women's aspirations to be 'good mothers' both antenatally and postnatally. Equally they should be reminded that postnatal depression is not necessarily a distinct postnatal event and can neither be viewed nor explained in purely postnatal terms.

WHAT ABOUT POSTNATAL CHOICE?

Jean Ball in 1995, reporting her study of reactions to motherhood highlighted that despite major changes in maternity care organisation and delivery of care

in delivery suites and neonatal units, the importar
unacknowledged and service provision under-res

First Class Delivery (noted that women made m
hospital postnatal services than any other aspect
it seems apparent, through the recent Healthcare
ongoing changes in maternity service delivery ha
this status quo.[17] Postnatal care, although acknowl
Services[2] and Maternity Matters,[3] generally rem
aims and objectives, and a serious omission in th
between women's expectations and desires for
received levels of support are clear in women's na
mother' narratives elucidate how the reality follov
tic notions of motherhood'. Women are not sup
physical and emotional demands of mothering
in women feeling exposed as 'bad mothers'. In la
reinforce the unsupportive nature of immediat
staff as largely absent and detrimental to a 'good
themselves as failures, which clearly impacts on

Women throughout pregnancy narrate an c
which invests them with a responsibility to be
This is a much more embodied responsibility t
to the nature of pregnancy as a physical and pl
women themselves can experience. However, v
in relegating fathers and actively seeking to ab
of good mothering. Following the birth of the
responsibility takes on a new dimension that i
baby. This is underpinned by the emotional di
often elusive in pregnancy, now informed by a
ure in their mothering abilities. Unlike pregna
were able to divest some responsibility to, ei
difficulties, or to hereditary factors, the mater
they provide postnatally renders them open
their mothering skills. Women are inherently
pregnancy the boundaries of normality have
much more ambiguous. The puerperium is tr
recovery from childbirth, but women feel they
independence and a return to non-pregnant wo
feeling *uncared for* and *uncared about*. Women re
and in breastfeeding which situates them as 'b
experts in the form of midwives promote breas

care as a domain of expertise and the language to which women themselves have access in order to express their emotional status.

EMOTIONAL STATUS AND CHOICE

Pregnancy is an acknowledged time of emotional lability for women, which endures into the postnatal period. Choice, although not unimportant to women, rather than facilitating desired experience often rather facilitates the necessity to conform to desired idealised identities. It is the failure to meet these identities that appears to mediate emotional distress and enduring psychological consequences rather than failures to fulfil a desired birth experience. This proffers a further explanation for the lack of effect that choice of care as a single variable has made to date with regard to psychological outcomes.[1,13] Emotional distress when it does occur is individualised, disparate and emerges from a multifaceted psychosocial matrix.

It seems imperative for the context of women's psychological health to be understood from a perspective that takes account of their entire maternity experience. The consumerist choice debate reinforced by policy, and academic and popular literature depicts choice in maternity care as increasing satisfaction with pregnancy and birth experiences, and thus directly contributing to emotional well-being.[14] For women who maintain normality and do not suffer any challenges to their desired birth experience, it seems that this may well be true. However, what is significant within women's subjective accounts is how offering choice can conversely render other women disempowered, guilty, angry and distressed. Women from the earliest point of contact are scrutinised under a defined framework of normality. Those who expect, yet fail to meet the normality criteria at any point in their pregnancies are labelled as abnormal and denied choice or charged with a remit of proving their normality before their choices can be fulfilled.

Unfulfilled choice, whilst seemingly, for some women, playing a contributory role to subsequent psychological sequelae, cannot be given the standing of a single causative factor. Women throughout their pregnancy strive to promote themselves as 'good mothers', act responsibly and make appropriate decisions. Many other discourses, influences and events serve to reinforce their status as 'good or bad mothers' throughout pregnancy. Women who maintain only a tenuous grasp of their 'good mother' identity are rendered emotionally vulnerable as pregnancy progresses. It seems apparent that those women who leave pregnancy emotionally vulnerable enter the postnatal period in the same state, regardless of delivery events. Postnatal events build on this level of emotional vulnerability, which appears to manifest in perceived failures to adequately fulfil 'good mother', 'gendered parenting' and 'domestic labourer' roles, perpetuating the descent into significant psychological distress.

For some women the location of emotional vulnerability is less apparent in their antenatal narratives, yet implicit in their postnatal accounts is a similar state of emotional vulnerability. This emerges from accounts of disappointing delivery experiences that did not meet with expectations and/or the overwhelming nature of being a 'real mother' characterised by loneliness, isolation and resentment. Many of these postnatal accounts are infused with some articulated loss of personal identity, as women feel constrained and pressured, in the postnatal period, by 'gendered parenting' and domestic labour roles. Resentment is articulated through narratives that compare female to male parenting roles. Whilst some women narrate an emotional vulnerability in the early postnatal period often as a result of individualised experiences, this emotional vulnerability does not manifest in enduring postnatal depression, suggesting that some women are equipped with better personal resources and are more empowered or enabled to restore personal identity than others. The differences among those women who narrated emotional distress and did not feel pushed to seek help and those who did, appears to be located in feelings of failure and inability to function rather than feelings of low mood. Those women pushed to seek help did so out of their perception of themselves as 'bad mothers' and an apparent inability to adequately fulfil idealised roles.

These accounts clearly illuminate a multifaceted image of postnatal depression. The privileged insight into postnatal depression that emerges from women's narratives appears to enable the conclusions that whilst women's accounts depict an individualised biography, they are underpinned by perceived failures to meet the idealised cultural and societal depictions that surround pregnancy and childbirth. There is no one consistent causative factor that characterises the experience of postnatal distress. The level of postnatal distress is perhaps mediated by personal resources, but is more clearly located in women's abilities to perform and perceive themselves as 'good mothers'. Hence, care givers need to be aware of the role they can play in women's aspirations to be 'good mothers' both antenatally and postnatally. Equally they should be reminded that postnatal depression is not necessarily a distinct postnatal event and can neither be viewed nor explained in purely postnatal terms.

WHAT ABOUT POSTNATAL CHOICE?

Jean Ball in 1995, reporting her study of reactions to motherhood highlighted that despite major changes in maternity care organisation and delivery of care in delivery suites and neonatal units, the importance of postnatal care remained unacknowledged and service provision under-resourced.

First Class Delivery (noted that women made more negative comments about hospital postnatal services than any other aspect of their maternity care[16] and it seems apparent, through the recent Healthcare Commission report, that the ongoing changes in maternity service delivery have failed to have an impact on this status quo.[17] Postnatal care, although acknowledged in the NSF for Maternity Services[2] and Maternity Matters,[3] generally remains less considered in policy aims and objectives, and a serious omission in the choice debate. Discrepancies between women's expectations and desires for support from care givers and received levels of support are clear in women's narratives. The 'babies create real mother' narratives elucidate how the reality following birth fails to meet 'romantic notions of motherhood'. Women are not supported by 'experts' to meet the physical and emotional demands of mothering following birth, which results in women feeling exposed as 'bad mothers'. In late postnatal narratives women reinforce the unsupportive nature of immediate postnatal care and implicate staff as largely absent and detrimental to a 'good mother' status, locating women themselves as failures, which clearly impacts on their sense of self-worth.

Women throughout pregnancy narrate an ownership of their pregnancies which invests them with a responsibility to be 'good mothers' to their fetuses. This is a much more embodied responsibility than that of fathers due in part to the nature of pregnancy as a physical and physiological event that only the women themselves can experience. However, women themselves are culpable in relegating fathers and actively seeking to absorb that responsibility as part of good mothering. Following the birth of the baby this individual sense of responsibility takes on a new dimension that involves the physical care of the baby. This is underpinned by the emotional dimension of mothering that was often elusive in pregnancy, now informed by a visible reality of success or failure in their mothering abilities. Unlike pregnancy and labour where women were able to divest some responsibility to, either, the fetus for problems or difficulties, or to hereditary factors, the materiality of the care and nurturing they provide postnatally renders them open to greater potential criticism of their mothering skills. Women are inherently conscious of this yet, whilst in pregnancy the boundaries of normality have been clear, postnatal norms are much more ambiguous. The puerperium is traditionally depicted as a time of recovery from childbirth, but women feel they are pushed too rapidly towards independence and a return to non-pregnant woman, which results in them often feeling *uncared for* and *uncared about*. Women report difficulties in providing care and in breastfeeding which situates them as 'bad mothers'. This occurs because experts in the form of midwives promote breastfeeding as the best thing for the baby and the thing that 'good mothers' do. Midwives, paradoxically, however, are cited by women as necessary and instrumental in achieving confidence and competence in caring for their babies. Hence midwives set the standards of good mothering but, due to lack of resource and the current system of service provision, they simultaneously provide insufficient care and support and position women as 'bad mothers'.

Lack of care reduces self worth by threatening the 'good mother' identity and engendering feelings of failure and guilt. Potential explanations for the discrepancies between expectation and receipt of care can be proffered by the assumed naturalness of mothering, the focus of maternity care on the well-being and safe delivery of the baby and the subsequent withdrawal of medical interest following that outcome as well as the often inadequate resourcing of postnatal services.

The results of this study have shown how personal and complex women's adjustment to motherhood is after birth. This highlights the need to focus attention on the individuality of women's experiences, particularly important when the mother is emotionally vulnerable due to factors or events over which she has no control. The skills and tools to recognise emotional vulnerability across the maternity spectrum alongside providing negotiated levels of individual care in the postnatal period would seem to be the key to identifying potential postnatal psychological distress. Psychological distress, however, is undeniably about how women themselves experience their pregnancies, relationships and individual events over the whole maternity period. Further, the way in which care is provided by midwives during the postnatal period has a clear and potentially enduring effect on women's emotional health. The failure to extend the consumerist model into the postnatal period appears to be a failure of the system to firstly fulfil its promise of choice and secondly an omission with consequences that unequivocally requires attention.

SUMMARY

Caregivers have the potential to make a significant difference to a woman's experience of childbirth regardless of her choices for care. This is likely to operate at many different levels, from the expert judgements that are made, the language that is used, how normality is presented, perceived and reinforced, how emotional vulnerability is recognised, understood and managed, to what extent women feel they are being cared for and cared about, supported, and able to make decisions affecting their care. Therefore, what an effective model of choice requires is a greater understanding, acknowledgement and respect of the complexity of how women understand and engage with not only their pregnancy, birth and postnatal experience, but with the care system and its providers.

Choice is clearly here to stay within the healthcare arena and invests care givers with a need to acknowledge choice with both integrity and responsibility. Models of care that offer choice need to be designed to take into consideration the dangers of offering choices that may not be fulfilled and of not extending choice into the postnatal environment. Foremost, however, choice needs to be presented within a realistic, open and honest forum that acknowledges choice, even within the current politicised health landscape, as a limited possibility. Women even as consumers, remain unequal partners as they struggle with a contemporary complexity of childbirth that involves the constraints of normalising discourses, their unique biographies, their potential vulnerability and the materiality of pregnancy and birth.

REFERENCES

1 Jomeen J, Martin CR. The impact of choice of maternity care on psychological health outcomes for women during pregnancy and the postnatal period. *J Eval Clin Pract.* 2008; **14**(3): 391–8.

2 Department of Health and Department of Education and Skills. *National Service Framework for Children, Young People and Maternity Services: Maternity Services.* London: Department of Health; 2004.

3 Department of Health. *Maternity Matters: choice, access and continuity of care in a safe service.* London: Department of Health; 2007.

4 House of Commons. *Health Committee Second Report. Session 1991–1992: Maternity Services.* London: HMSO; 1992.

5 Gatrell C. *Hard Labour: the sociology of parenthood.* Maidenhead: Open University Press; 2005.

6 Oakley A. *From Here to Maternity: becoming a mother.* Harmondsworth: Penguin; 1981.

7 Ohman SG, Grunewald C, Waldenstrom U. Women's worries during pregnancy: testing the Cambridge Worries Scale on 200 Swedish women. *Scand J Caring Sci.* 2003; **17**: 148–52.

8 Statham H, Green J, Kafetsios K. Who worries that something might be wrong with the baby? A prospective study of 1072 women. *Birth.* 1997; **24**(4): 223–33.

9 Lowe NK. Self efficacy for labour and childbirth fears in nulliparous pregnant women. *J Psychosom Obst Gynaecol.* 2000; **21**(4): 219–24.

10 Green J, Baston H. Feeling in control during labour: concepts, correlates and consequences. *Birth.* 2003; **30**(4): 235–47.

11 Mander R. Who chooses the choices? *Modern Midwife.* 1993; **3**(1): 23–5.

12 Weaver J. Childbirth. In: Ussher JM, editor. *Women's Health: contemporary international health perspectives.* Leicester: The British Psychological Society; 2000.

13 Renfrew MJ, Green JM, Spiby H. *Evidence submitted to the House of Commons Health Committee Maternity Sub-committee 1st inquiry (2003:03).* Mother and Infant Research Unit: University of Leeds.

14 Hodnett ED, Downe S, Edwards N, *et al.* Home-like versus conventional institutional setting for birth. *The Cochrane Library.* 2005; **3**.

15 Ball J. *Reactions to Motherhood: the role of postnatal care.* 2nd ed. Hale: Books for Midwives Press; 1995.

16 Audit Commission. *First Class Delivery: improving maternity services in England and Wales.* London: Audit Commission Publications; 1997.

17 Healthcare Commission. *Towards Better Births: a review of maternity services in England.* London: Healthcare Commission; 2008.

Index